Praise for *A Real Woman's Guide to a Fabulous Body*

"I have this new found freedom like someone has broken the chains and released me from the prison of dieting hell!"
– Rebecca, Victoria

"If you want to lose weight without dieting or missing out on the good things in life, I highly recommend this book! I never knew how easy it could be to lose the weight and feel amazing. After all the diets and hard work that got me nowhere in the past, it was such a relief to find the simple solution. It's easy to read, easy to follow and identifies untold links to great health. Thank you, Julie, for your words of wisdom and the great results! I can now focus on other achievements, knowing I will always maintain this great health – in mind and body."
– Sally, Victoria

"Thank you, Julie, for your brilliant advice and great results! I wouldn't have got to where I am today without your book, and I am very grateful for that. And who would have thought I would be in a book about MY weight loss Thank you!! You Rock!!!!!"
– Donna, Victoria

"Thank you for inspiring a lazy Mum!! We have just finished having our first fresh juice session and it was all gone in 2 seconds flat! And the yummy soup passed the test last night! The family also had a bit of a think tank about how we could prepare healthier options for the young boys' dinners after I showed my husband the scary ingredients in chicken nuggets! You do a brilliant job of making a big difference in people's lives. "
– Anna, Queensland

For copies of this book and information about programs:

w: www.foodfix.com.au and e: info@foodfix.com.au

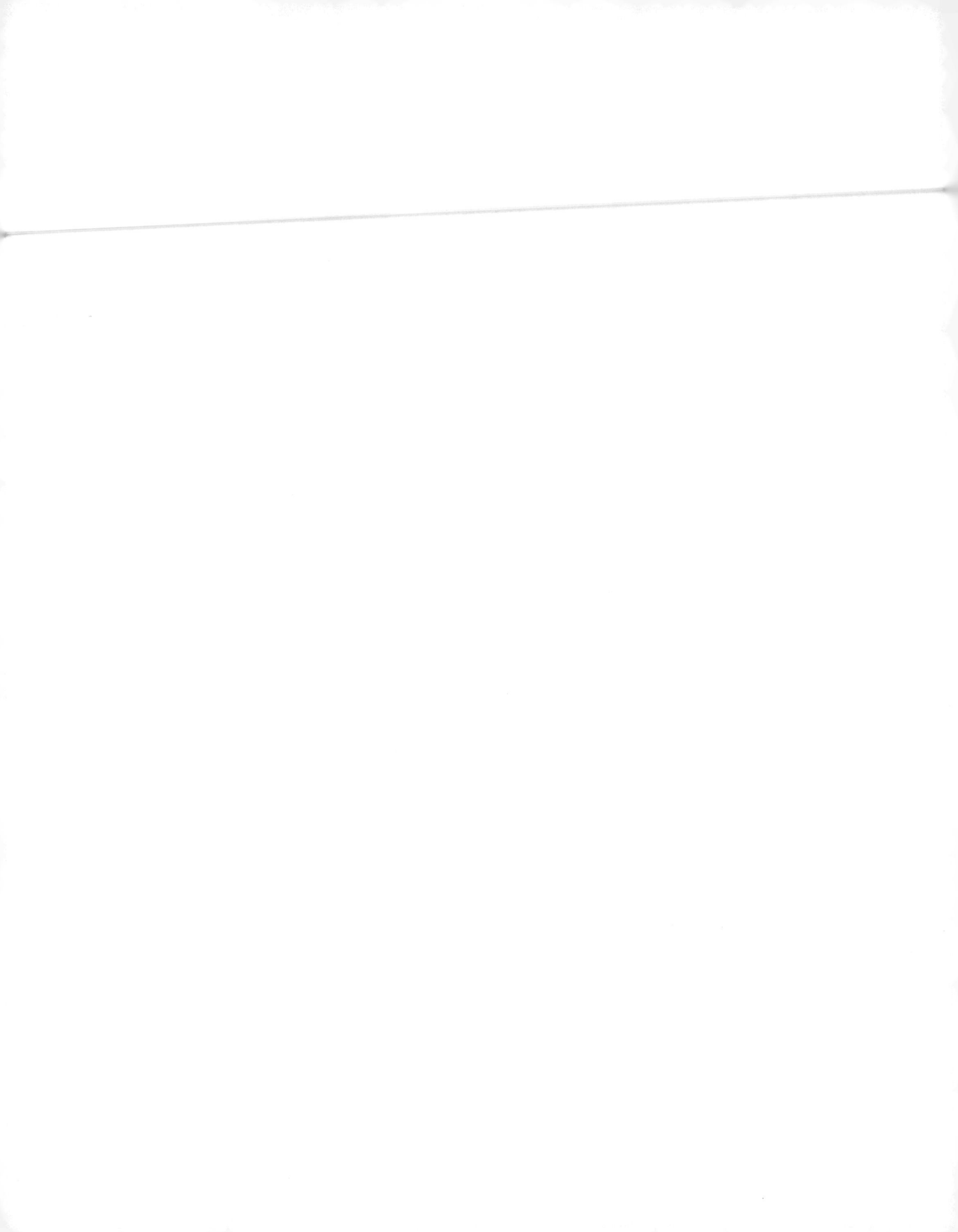

A Real Woman's Guide to a Fabulous Body

We lost weight and you can too

By
Julie Regan

A Real Woman's Guide to a Fabulous Body
Author – Julie Regan

www.foodfix.com.au
julie@foodfix.com.au

Editing by Alex Mitchell www.AuthorSupportServices.com

Typesetting by Master Page Design

Cover design by Casey Nee

Photography by Jarrod Barnes

Printed and bound by Create Space - www.createspace.com

National Library of Australia Cataloguing-in-Publication
Regan, Julie
A Real Woman's Guide to a Fabulous Body: We lost weight and you can too
1st edition.
978-0-9872279-2-8 (pbk.)
Weight loss
Health
Self-actualization (Psychology)
Dewey Number: 613.712

Dedication

I dedicate this book to the beautiful women
who have inspired me to tell their stories.

Acknowledgements

Thank you to Sally, a wonderful student, friend and mentor! You have inspired me along my journey.

To Damian, a naturopath, kinesiologist and personal trainer extraordinaire. Your words and methods keep me well.

Thank you to my wonderful editor and advisor, Alex Mitchell, who has great vision and was quick to understand exactly what was in my head!

And to my wonderful husband, Craig, thank you for your relentless support, love, advice and belief in me.

Preface

Real, everyday women… the penny dropped!

After many years in the nutrition and fitness industry, meeting countless women trying everything possible to lose weight and get fit, I had found the answer.

I realised how real, everyday women could offer so much more hope, advice and support than any gym advert or expert opinion. Ordinary women, who had been overweight, unhealthy and lost, yet had found their way to success, were the people best qualified to show others what was possible, what was REAL.

So I listened, interviewed and travelled the path alongside these inspiring women and can now share their secrets – as well as mine – with you.

The stories are of women who achieved great success in body and mind – despite life and other obstacles getting in the way. It amazes me how courageous they have been to publically declare they needed help to become strong, confident and successful women.

Together, we discovered the ingredients that had been missing to create weight loss and health success. Each woman found their own missing piece of the puzzle - mindset, eating, exercise, planning, and overcoming obstacles. Once the pieces fell into place, every one of these real, average women suddenly found that it *was* possible to eat delicious food and enjoy exercising. Each one reached her goal weight and along with it, the health and vitality that had been eluding her.

What a pleasure it has been to see these ladies, who were once unhappy and lacking in confidence, transform their lives and achieve great health and fabulous bodies. To travel the journey with these women as they succeeded in getting the life they so dearly wanted has been the most satisfying achievement in my life (apart from my children, of course!).

These ordinary women have enabled me to understand the most difficult of challenges we face when trying to losing weight; the keys to getting started, what motivates women to stay on track and how to enjoy the journey.

Donna, Sally, Liz, Jen and Jade share their stories with you and lead you on a wonderful, supportive journey, one where you will feel a connection with the common issues stopping you from losing weight, and find the answers YOU need to enjoy great health and a great body.

They have achieved their dreams, and have all said to me in their own way:

"If I can do it, any woman can."

Contents

Introduction

We live in confusing times, times when we are bombarded with constant messages about how to achieve perfect health and perfect bodies. The answers to all our questions and problems appear to be easily solved, if we just follow the advice of this person or that magazine.

So we believe the promises and do as we are told, full of hope. But somehow, the amazing figure and vibrant good health does not materialise, and we find ourselves in the same place or even a worse position. In failure, we try something new, only to fail again. Slowly, we become uncertain. We doubt ourselves and our self-esteem becomes lower. We start to believe we will never be able to achieve our health goals and dreams, and eventually resign ourselves to defeat.

Well the good news is, things are about to change in your life…

Welcome to your new healthy world

Imagine this:

You wake up feeling energised and enthusiastic about the day ahead. Your mood is bright and you're ready to take on the world. You enjoy getting dressed, as your clothes fit beautifully and your skin is glowing. After a tasty breakfast, your focus is crystal clear and you stay that way for the whole day. You achieve more than you ever used to – with energy and drive. You deal with a couple of difficult tasks which used to put you in a bad mood, but now you find yourself calm and capable of dealing with anything.

When the kids get home from school, you play football and have running races. Exhilarated, you organise homework and a healthy dinner and still have the focus and energy to finish making those last business calls and emails for the day. By 8pm, you sit down for a chat with your husband about your day and you look forward to the next…..

What an amazing life you are living!

Now, coming back to the present, how do you currently feel each day? Does this scenario sound more familiar…..

Your day begins as you wake up feeling exhausted and dreading all the tasks that lay ahead. You hate getting dressed, as nothing fits well and you curse your body. You grab a sugary cereal and coffee to get you moving. You're tired by 3pm and say "No" to the kids when they ask you to play in the garden. You watch a bit of TV and fall into bed at night, exhausted.

And perhaps you have tried every diet and exercise program that comes along, without success. Maybe you see other people eating exactly what you are eating, and losing weight, but you are staying the same size. So why aren't you successful, you wonder?

Because a piece of the puzzle has been missing, preventing you from achieving what you know you can achieve with your body. Hidden amongst the stories of these six everyday women, you will find your answers and the key that fits for you.

These ladies demonstrate that it's possible for *anyone* to lose fat, feel great and achieve the body of their dreams. Like you, they were ready for something better, but just didn't know where to begin. Armed with the right information and guidance, they have changed their lives forever. Follow their lead and you will discover your own key to success, with a life of vitality and health. A life where food is a joy and your body reflects the balance you have found.

You will be guided every step of the way as you move towards your new life. You will discover how important it is to free your mind from any past failures, and how to really set goals that suit YOU. You'll learn how to get prepared, how to stock your pantry, how to eat, when to eat, how to exercise less for better results and how to remove any barriers to achieving the body you want. You will discover the strategies the women in this book have implemented, to create a healthy new life for yourself – a life where it's easy to stay in shape and feel great, forever.

You do have the power to change and live the life of your dreams. We all have a special key that unlocks the door to our path of success. Once you make a few simple changes, you will realise that you can do *anything you want* with your health *and* your body.

YOU can change your body and your health; you just need support, guidance and the *right* knowledge. It's easy, and it's about things you already know, as well as the basics you will soon discover. Your common sense has been guiding you in the right direction; you just need a little encouragement and reinforcement from women like yourself…

Understanding the Big Picture

24 Years: 66kg

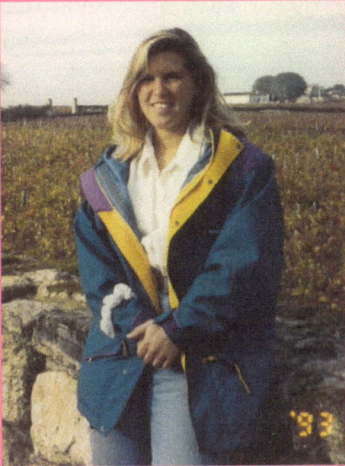

35 Years: 63kg

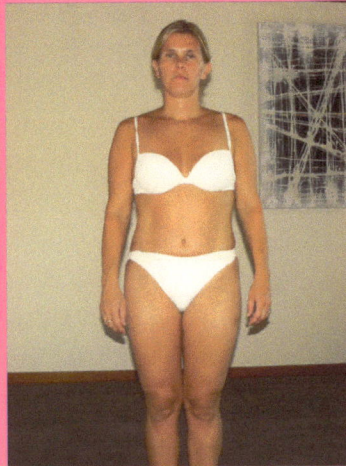

41 Years: 56kg

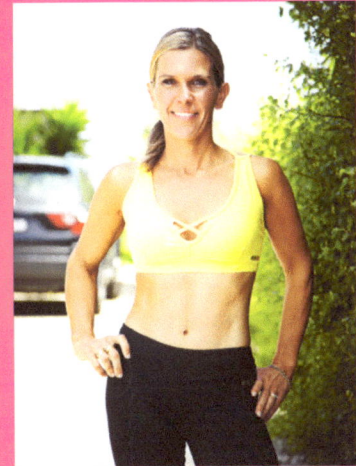

"The great breakthrough in your life comes when you realise that you can learn anything you need to learn to accomplish any goal that you set for yourself. This means there are no limits on what you can be, have or do"

-Brian Tracy

MY STORY

Julie, 41, mother of two, nutritionist and personal trainer

One day I woke up fat…

Growing up, I loved sport and all things physical. From the age of eight, I remember the thrill I felt as I ran around the Little Athletics track. So it seemed natural to find a career that involved the physical.
At the age of 21, I completed my Physical Education Degree and secured a job in a fitness club, ready to help the members with my new-found knowledge. I soon discovered the number one reason people had for joining the gym was to lose weight. Many said they wanted to get fit too, but it ran a distant second place to losing weight.

I kept very fit and thought I had all the answers to maintaining a lean body. However, within two years of starting the job, I was horrified to discover that I was fat. It seemed to happen overnight. And the scary part was I had no idea how it happened. I thought that with my level of fitness and eating habits it just wasn't possible. I started to doubt myself - how could I help others if I couldn't help myself? And how did the average woman stand a chance if *I* couldn't do it? I realised I actually didn't have all the answers and still had a lot to learn.

I could certainly help people improve their training technique, improve their fitness and give them an idea of healthy food choices, but I had little success with real and permanent weight loss for myself or my clients.

3

So I threw myself into learning, working in health promotion, training as an exercise physiologist and also becoming a personal trainer. I mostly learnt that I didn't know much, and for a while that was very disheartening. I did slowly lose my excess weight, but I wasn't the lean machine I wanted to be – not yet.

At 25, I began to experiment with my diet and that of others and began to understand that food was the major factor preventing success. This led me to Post Graduate studies in nutrition and with this, another phase of thinking I knew everything. I was seeing client after client in my business, but even with my newly acquired qualification, I just kept *telling them what to eat*.

I had seen a number of nutritionists, dieticians and naturopaths in relation to my own health and weight and they all did the same thing I was doing – hand out lists of foods to eat and foods to avoid.

The word 'avoid' seemed irritating yet alluring to me. My compliance time for these restrictive diets was around one week, and I was a person who was highly motivated! So how could I expect my clients to achieve their goals with this technique if I couldn't do it myself?

This was my 'light bulb' moment, when the penny dropped and I finally worked out what it was I needed to do – I needed to DO THINGS DIFFERENTLY! Before I could truly help others, I had to find the missing ingredient (excuse the pun) to permanent results without dieting. So I changed my whole approach – with remarkable results.

This is where my journey of self-discovery began. I developed a new strategy, one that recognised we are all complex human beings, and we all require much more than just an eating plan and a training program. I looked at the big picture – the mind and the body, life and all its challenges. I realised that what I needed when I was 20 was very different to my needs at 30. Using myself as a guinea pig, I began to consider what was missing in the big picture and preventing me from achieving my goals successfully. My self-analysis revealed I was missing a clear vision, as well as goal

MY STATS		
	BEFORE	**AFTER**
Weight:	63kg	56kg
Dress Size:	12	8
Time from fat to fab: 12 weeks		
Key to success: Seeing the big picture		

setting and preparation. I decided that if I could fill in each of these missing pieces, I would be on my way to achieving my goals.

Armed with a solid plan, I began by creating a vision and a list of goals, writing out my dreams and then living as if I had achieved them already - every day. I saw myself as a fit, lean personal trainer, exuding vitality. I worked on being prepared, and became as organised as possible in my daily routine in order to stick to my mission. I wrote down all the obstacles and issues I could foresee and counteracted them with a potential list of solutions.

Within a few months, I was fit and lean. I looked and lived like a personal trainer. This began a six year period during which I was in great shape and in perfect health. And at last I had great success helping clients achieve similar results, by helping them to see the big picture too.

However, things changed for me once again when I started my family. My priorities changed with my new lifestyle and my own health suffered. After my first baby was born, I found myself with 22kg to lose. Once again, I put in place the steps to lose the weight. I created a plan to improve my diet and fitness level and got back the body I wanted within months. The birth of my second child, however, bought with it a new set of challenges.

I was 35 when I sprained my pelvis while in labour with my daughter. I spent the next three months wheelchair-bound, which was a traumatic time. I couldn't walk, and couldn't even lift my baby without help. I had a very busy two-year-old boy who needed his mum, and a husband who was working long hours in our restaurant and catering business.

Trying to manage two small children without being able to walk or drive took its toll. Food became my best friend and I gave up any attempt to remain healthy. I was drinking more wine in an attempt to cope, wasn't getting enough sleep with the usual challenges that come with small children and struggled through each day. I hit rock bottom, both physically and mentally. This is where the complex nature of the human mind really became clear for me.

The turning point came one day when I looked in the mirror and saw someone I didn't know or like. I had gained a lot of weight, and at 63kg I looked 45 rather than 35. I cried for two hours before deciding it was time to get my life and body back.

I went back to my holistic health plan and once again got my body and health back into top condition. Even under such trying circumstances, I saw that the strategy of getting my mindset right and looking for the missing ingredient was effective. I hit my target of 56kg in 12 weeks and was able to maintain it for the next five years. Then another challenge presented itself to test my resilience and skills.

At the age of 40 I fell down the stairs in the middle of the night and broke a bone in my foot. I was frustrated and in pain, but soon my thoughts turned to how this would impact my body. I knew I had to think ahead and plan for my recovery in order to avoid weight gain and end up blaming my injury for it.

I was able to do rehabilitation exercises to maintain strength and tone in my lower body, and continued with training my upper body. With time, I included swimming and bike riding.

I reminded myself how easy it had been to eat without any awareness and suffer the consequences of weight and fat gain. So my number one priority was to maintain good eating habits. I made a concerted effort to eat well during my convalescence, and over the next four months I was pleased that my size remained the same.

The key to my success was in understanding the big picture. I had learnt the importance of assessing each part of the equation and focussing my energy on the missing pieces. To get results I had to have the right mindset, make sure I was prepared with my food, and do the right type of exercise.

Each time I needed to take action, I broke down my goals into bite size pieces. My goals were:

1. To develop a lean, fat free body
2. To attain a high level of fitness
3. To provide inspiration to others as someone who had 'been there'.

1. Develop a lean, fat free body

- I took a 'before' photo and measurements to provide me with something to measure down the track. I then put this data out of my mind, as it represented the past. I diarised dates of when I wanted to achieve my goals, but my mind was mainly focused on feeling great, eating well and enjoying the journey.
- I decided to keep my eating plan simple. I didn't want to be overwhelmed with the enormity of the task ahead. I looked for easy recipes or foods I could combine simply to create a healthy meal.
- I wrote out a healthy eating weekly menu, including snacks, and then bought everything I needed from the butcher, market, health food store and supermarket.
- I threw out or gave away all the food that did not fit my healthy eating criteria, and gave the pantry, fridge and freezer a good clean out. When I restocked with healthy foods I loved to eat, I stacked them neatly so that everything was easy to find and tempting to eat.
- I bought a snack pack to transport my healthy meals and snacks when I was out of the house or working.
- I cooked extra food such as chicken and roast vegetables for the next day's meals. This eliminated the pressure of having to prepare something from scratch for every meal.

- I began eating mindfully and regularly – when my body needed fuelling. This way, I knew I would never feel hungry or deprived and it allowed me to maintain a positive state of mind. It gave me great comfort to know I would just eat the next time I was hungry!
- I reinforced my successes and focused on how great I was feeling – and starting to look. This served as enormous motivation to keep me on track.

2. Attain a high level of fitness

- Measurable fitness goals helped me keep focused. I entered myself and a friend in a fun run six months ahead. This gave me a specific timeline to improve my running fitness.
- I worked out a training program which included weights, running and interval training. I reviewed this every month for six months. I recorded my running times and weight sessions to ensure I was progressing.

3. Provide inspiration to others as someone who had 'been there'

- The point of difference I had for my clients was that rather than being a young fit trainer who simply loves to exercise, I had also lived the life of someone overweight and unhealthy. I had been there and back four times.
- I had learned how to overcome obstacles with focus, resilience and a positive mind in order to maintain the body I want.
- I knew how complex weight loss and fitness could be, so I could relate to all the lost and disheartened women I met. Sharing my stories helped them to realise they too could change their bodies and change their lives; they just needed to find their missing key.

The Missing Ingredient

Do you find yourself searching for that missing key to your weight loss dreams? Does the new buzz phrase or diet have you searching the internet or hitting the magazine stands with the hope that THIS will be the answer to your weight loss prayers?

Sometimes, the important elements needed for successful health and a toned body can be missed through paying too much attention to irrelevant or even minor details.

On the journey towards better health, you will have formed your own opinions on what works, what doesn't, how much fat to eat or how much exercise to do. You may have tried many strategies: eating more, eating less, a new diet or training program. It is tempting to think that doing one thing and doing it properly will be the answer to losing those magical kilos or successfully running a marathon. But usually, it isn't.

Like many people, you may have suspected there are some OTHER reasons you are not achieving the results you want. Let's consider some of those reasons. Firstly, you are unique, with your own individual set of experiences. Every day of your life you have experienced, learnt and even eaten differently to others around you. You have had your own illnesses, injuries, stresses and hurdles. You may have been on diets, or perhaps you have never exercised in your life. Your mindset is unique and you have your own triggers that motivate you in life.

Secondly, you have a certain level of knowledge about strategies for health and weight loss. You may have completed formal studies or gathered your knowledge via friends and the media. Once you have gathered all the *right* information, you can discover YOUR missing link. A degree does not guarantee all the answers, and the media is not always accurate!

No one else can tell you exactly how to achieve all of your dreams. Having the right information will give you some guidance and provide you with healthy choices, but only you can make those choices and decide what is going to work for you.

Finally, it's time to start trusting your intuition, the voice that guides you in the right direction – the one that reminds you that a fad diet won't work and an extra class at the gym won't help you drop a dress size. The voice that says diet soft drink doesn't make sense and that excuses are holding you back. You have heard this voice many times, so listen to it and remember that your common sense and intuition are always right.

To find the solution you need for success in health and fat loss, you will need to open your mind to all the factors that may have put you in the situation you are in today. Ask yourself, "How did I get where I am today?"

Keep your mind open to the experiences and ideas you read. Look for the missing ingredient that lies within one of the stories or strategies. As you read through the personal stories and circumstances, perhaps a particular woman will resonate with you. You may feel a connection or a common thread which aligns your story to theirs.

In some way or another, we all have the same story. As you read through the strategies and complete the action plans you will learn, understand and unveil your own answers to a healthy, happy life.

Think about the big picture from an impartial perspective, as if you are looking in from the outside, and let the learning REALLY begin.

Action

Mind...
Keep in mind that there are thousands of women in your shoes today; women who want to change their lives. You just need the right information to take the action that is right for you. Believe that you CAN do it and open your mind.

Body...
Think about the body you want – how you want your body to feel and look for the rest of your life. Hold that image in your mind each day.

Food...
Forget your old thoughts on eating for health and fat loss. Forget about fad diets and anything that doesn't have you focused on healthy eating. Start with a blank canvas and begin adding to it. Surround yourself with healthy, knowledgeable people, whether they are nutritionists, health experts, athletes, mothers or friends; search for those oozing vitality and sound knowledge - and start learning.

Free Your Mind

"Change has a considerable psychological impact on the human mind.

To the fearful it is threatening because it means that things may get worse.

To the hopeful it is encouraging because things may get better.

To the confident it is inspiring because the challenge exists to make things better"

-King Whitney Jr.

DONNA'S STORY

Donna, 37, mother of three, student

Once I realised I *could* lose the weight, you couldn't stop me!

Before kids, Donna had a successful career in insurance. She loved the feeling of achievement that came with helping people through her work. She was talented in her field and clients often congratulated and thanked her for providing exceptional service. The recognition from others, and her own belief in her abilities, meant Donna was a confident and happy woman. She rarely doubted herself and believed she could achieve any goal she'd set.

Before: 90kg

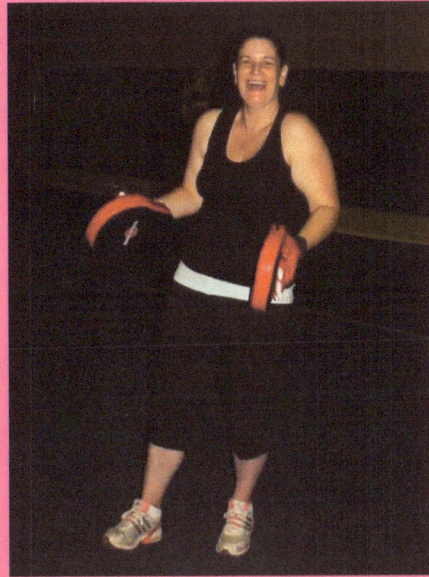

After: 68kg

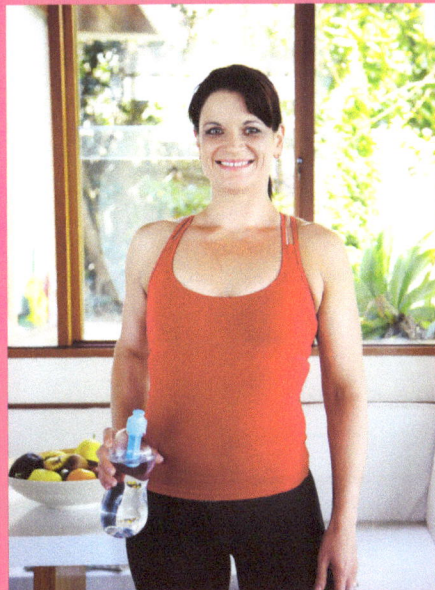

At 30 years of age, Donna left the workforce to start a family. As she settled into her new role, she found that although she loved being a mum, she felt somewhat incomplete. Focusing on the needs of her family and struggling to find enough time for her own needs, bit by bit, Donna felt she was losing her sense of identity. She began to feel lost and out of control of her life.

By the time baby number three was born five years later, Donna weighed 90kg and had begun to think she would never get her body back. She had always been so proud of her ability to believe in herself and achieve anything, yet now her confidence was at an all-time low and her weight was at an all-time high. It was a horrible feeling for Donna – she was unhappy and disappointed in herself for losing control of her healthy body and mind.

Donna realised she had to take action if she wanted things to change. And she certainly did want change; she'd had enough of feeling overweight and depressed.

Donna began her journey back to health by getting some guidance at the gym. She worked hard to re-establish her sense of worth and self-belief. She stopped listening to the self-talk that was telling her she couldn't lose the weight and starting focusing on strategies and goals to get results. Donna changed her mindset to focus on what she COULD do, rather than what she couldn't.

Her self-talk changed to "I can" and "I will", and this cleared her mind of the mental obstacles she had been carrying around. The sense of relief was overwhelming, and she found it freed her to be able to focus on DOING. Her next step was to change her eating habits, and her confidence grew as the weight started to fall off. As Donna achieved each of her goals, she felt her self-belief return bit by bit and her self-confidence soared. Her goals were to:

1. Lose 20kg and three dress sizes
2. Have more energy
3. Improve her moods
4. Run 10km
5. Feel brilliant!

DONNA'S STATS		
	BEFORE	AFTER
Weight:	90kg	68kg
Dress Size:	16	12
Time from fat to fab: 6 months		
Key to success: Believing in myself		

I asked Donna some questions about her journey

Tell us about the moment you decided to change your body and your health.

"During my third pregnancy, I put on a great deal of weight. It was when my baby was three months old that I realised I was not losing the excess weight from the pregnancy. I was embarrassed to bump into people I knew, so I started avoiding leaving the house as I didn't want people to see me. The day I saw the dreaded 90kg on the scales, I knew I was in a place I did not want to be. I distinctly remember the thought running through mind: *"How did I get here?"*

I knew if I didn't do something to change my situation, it was really going to have a terrible effect on my health and life, forever."

What thoughts initially stopped you from believing you could achieve your dreams?

"I had always maintained a healthy weight before having children, so I was shocked to find myself so overweight after my third child. I lost confidence in myself and wondered if I was ever going to be able to get my body back to the way I wanted it. I thought I would be chasing that dream forever without ever achieving it. I didn't like thinking that way."

How did you get started?

"I began by asking myself some questions: Where do I want to be? What do I want to achieve? What are my options? Who can I enlist to help me on my new pathway?

The first step I took was to look to experts for guidance.

I rejoined the local gym and asked the staff there for advice on training and nutrition."

How did you overcome your lack of self-belief?

"I enlisted a coach and we began by working out my goals and dreams. As we began to map out my goals, it became apparent that I didn't actually believe I could achieve them! I was saying things like, "I tried to lose the baby fat but couldn't do it", and "I would like to run 10km, but I don't think I can." The funny thing is, I didn't even realise my self-belief was so low until I uttered those words."

"If you think you can or you think you can't, you are always right"
Henry Ford

WOW, such negative self-talk Donna was carrying around! It was one of those moments where suddenly everything made sense – she had her 'light bulb moment' and realised why she wasn't making progress with her weight loss. Her mind was making change impossible!

This honesty enabled Donna to see how her inner talk was hindering her progress and preventing her from achieving her goals. Bringing her thoughts into the open allowed Donna to address her self-doubt and change her way of thinking. She then felt free to take on her challenges with confidence, and with each small success, her belief in herself became stronger and her commitment more concrete.

She thought back to times she was fit and lean and felt like a million dollars, and began to focus on that image. With a fresh outlook, Donna began writing down her goals and started *seeing herself* every day as a trim, fit and healthy woman. These revelations allowed Donna to clear her mind and she was ready for action.

"What you focus on becomes your reality"
Lee Milteer

What was the first strategy you implemented?

"After getting my mindset right, I knew the most important thing I needed to change was how I was eating, so that became my focus and I began to implement a whole new way of eating."

What kept you on track when you felt like giving up?

"When I realised I *could* achieve any goal, I kept looking at the bigger goals I had for myself. Having the end in mind helped to keep me focused. I saw myself as I wanted to be and it kept me headed in the right direction. There didn't seem to be any other alternative future in my mind.

Once I *decided* I was really going to achieve my goals, I never felt like giving up. If I wandered off track for a day, I just got back to it the following day."

What advice do you have for a woman who wants to change her body?

"Don't ever think you can't do it. Recall a time when you did achieve success with your body, no matter how small, and hold onto that image. And remember that thousands of women have been in the same place as you and have gone on to achieve success by believing in themselves.

Set achievable goals for yourself and go for it. Having the goal of running 10km gave me a tangible goal, and I found a fun run to enter so I could set my goal date around an event day. Running isn't for everyone, so choose fitness goals that suit you, such as swimming 2km, walking the Kokoda Trail, riding or competing in a team event. And set goals with your eating habits. If you are committed to it 100%, you will achieve anything you set out to achieve – especially if you have made a financial commitment!"

Within six months, Donna had lost 16kg and decided to keep going. She was happy to continue using her strategies, as they were working! She was eating a healthy diet and continued to experience success by dropping a further 6kg and achieving some great fitness goals. Next, she completed a 14km fun run and was stronger than ever. She felt fantastic and had a renewed, healthy relationship with food and her mind.

Donna then set her eyes on helping others to achieve their dreams. She started a personal training course and began sharing her story to inspire others. She was already acting – and therefore living – as a teacher, helper and personal trainer.

Donna had stopped constantly worrying about food and her weight, and was free to live her life.

Beliefs and Believing

Change Your Mind

How many times have you heard that niggling little voice in your head saying "I am trying hard, but I'll never look how I want to look", or "I'll try to lose weight, but I know it won't work"? By listening to these words you are giving them the power to control your actions. This is negative reinforcement – you are focusing on what you DON'T want instead of what you DO want. Whatever you say often enough with strong conviction is what you will get.

Many women fail to achieve their health goals because they haven't changed their minds. They may change their behaviour in the short term, but they are subconsciously waiting for it to be over so they can get back to living their 'real' life. This is very common with fad diets. Once it is over and the normal diet resumes, the weight comes straight back on and it reinforces that success is impossible. This cycle can lead to a path of self-destruction, where women mentally beat themselves up for their supposed lack of willpower for the rest of their lives.

You must believe before you can achieve

Think about what has stopped you from thinking you can achieve the body and health you want. Do you make excuses or listen to voices in your head telling you that you will fail? Perhaps you blame other people or family members who have not supported you? Ask yourself: "What thoughts are holding me back?"

Start believing you *can* achieve your goals. You must unreservedly commit to that belief, otherwise you will subconsciously take action to ensure you never get there. Find a way to believe in yourself; stop *pretending* you do and make it your reality. The minute you decide to change things and start believing you can do anything, you will be filled with a sense of power and your self-esteem will improve immediately. You will find clarity and your motivation will kick in.

We are in control of every thought, decision and action we take

Be Emotional

Emotions are a great tool for bringing about change. They allow your dreams to become vivid and alive in your mind. The more you feel your desires in your head, the more real they become. Adrenaline kicks in and your subconscious starts to believe your dreams are your reality.

Change Your Labels

People label themselves, sometimes without even knowing they do it. They refer to themselves or to others with adjectives that either make them feel better or worse about themselves. Are you labelling yourself in a positive or negative light? What words do you use to describe yourself? If you use words like 'fat', 'hopeless', 'failure' or 'unworthy', remove these from your vocabulary. They are very destructive to your self-esteem and will hold you back from achieving your goals. Banish them from your life forever and only use words about yourself that describe how you aspire to be.

Labels are only good if they make you feel better about yourself

Start thinking of yourself as a winner, an achiever; someone who is full of confidence, energy and positivity. Try describing yourself with these labels: 'a healthy role model', 'an athlete', 'a fit and fabulous female', a 'success'. You are all these things already; you just may not have found them in yourself yet. These words will become who you are, your identity, so choose whatever feels comfortable to you. Imagine people referring to you in this way. As you begin to believe it, and make the appropriate changes in your life, people *will* begin to think of you with these adjectives. Think how good you will feel about yourself when that happens!

Fake It Till You Make It

Surround yourself with like-minded, goal orientated people who add to your sense of self-belief, understand your journey, inspire, educate and offer you valuable advice and support. As you mix with these people, you will slowly start to act like them, and as you execute this role, you will become the person you want to be. It will begin to feel normal to do inspiring things, strive for your goals and follow your dreams.

If others are doing it, you can too

It's time to start believing in yourself and your ability to achieve anything you set your mind to. Do it with complete honesty – truthfully and instinctively believe in yourself. Change your mind, imagine yourself already there, ignore the negative voices, listen to successful people and get started!

Action

Mind...

Consider where you are right now versus where you want to be. If you were to view yourself from a distance, what would you see? Would you see someone with the confidence to go after what she wants? Would you see her achieving goals and moving forward with her plans? Or would you see someone who falters, makes excuses and hides from the challenges of achievement?

Try this exercise to find a different perspective:

Sit in a comfortable chair, close your eyes and take three deep breaths. Imagine yourself at a fork in a road. There are two roads leading in different directions.

The road to the left takes you on a path where nothing has changed. Walk for a while down this road, and think of yourself one year from now, still in the same place in your life you are now.

See yourself doing the same things as you are now and imagine how you feel and look. You have gained a few extra kilos; you feel sluggish and unhappy about your health. Then think about yourself 5, 10 and 20 years from now, when still nothing has changed. How do you look and feel? Probably heavier and unhappier, suffering from a number of ailments and a huge case of weariness. You look older than you are and you certainly feel it.

Now go back to the fork in the road. Imagine yourself taking the pathway to the right, the one that leads to a life of eating well and exercising regularly.

Imagine yourself one year from now. You look radiantly healthy and younger than your age. You feel brilliant – totally relaxed and healthy. You are a role model to your family and friends and it is so easy for you to maintain your new state of health. You love your new life and could never return to the old, unhappy you. People comment on how well you look, how much younger you seem, how you are filled with endless energy and a great attitude. You have an air of confidence; you are a woman who looks like she rises to the challenge. You look happy and capable of achieving anything.

Thinking back, which path would you prefer to take? The path of change may seem difficult at first, but *not* changing your direction will cause you even more problems as time goes on.

When you go to bed tonight, close your eyes and repeat this activity. Add lots of details to the scenes in your mind and include as much emotion as you can muster. These emotions of excitement, satisfaction and achievement will provide further clarity and motivation and allow your mind to see this picture as real.

This is the new you, so start believing. Once you begin down the path of change, you will feel better – every single day for the rest of your life.

Body...

Take a photo of yourself in bathers. See yourself as you truly are right now. It's time to stop pretending that you are something different and see the reality. This action will demonstrate that you are ready to face the truth. It will be there in full colour. As you look back on this photo in time, you will see how far you have come since you began your journey.

Now that you have your 'before' shot, you can stop focusing on where you began, and look to the future. Focus on what you want, not on what you don't want.

Next, create an 'after' shot. This might be a photo of you when you were at your ideal weight or even a photo of your head on your 'ideal' body from a magazine. Just as the athlete visualises herself winning the race, see yourself in your new body. Focus on this image with all your emotion and enjoy the feeling. This is your destiny, so begin living as this person from this moment on.

Believe you are the 'after' photo from this moment on, all day and all night. To remind yourself who you are becoming, place a copy of the 'after' shot all around the house, in your diary or as your screensaver.

Food...

Get started by changing at least two current habits. Choose changes in behaviours or actions that you know your mind and lifestyle can manage. That way you will maintain these changes, they will become *normal* in your daily life and you will experience a feeling of success. You will feel better within a week and may start noticing some changes in your body, too.

Cut out	Two food types you can manage without
	e.g. sugar and fast food
Take up	Two healthy habits
	e.g. daily walking and drinking more water

Discover your Goals and Dreams

Before: 70kg

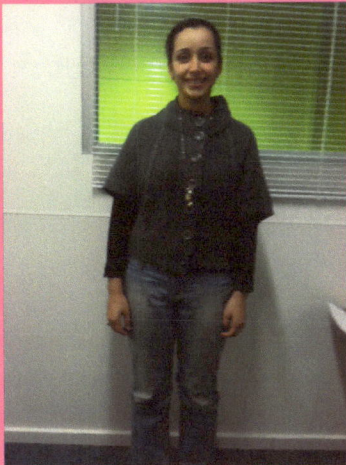

20 weeks: 59kg

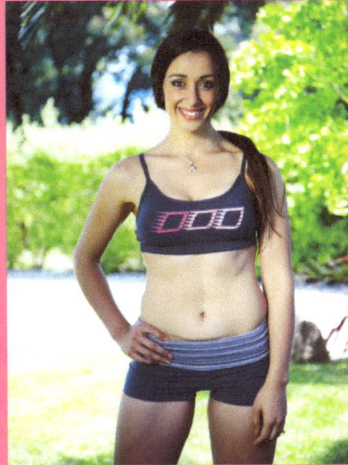

32 weeks: 56kg

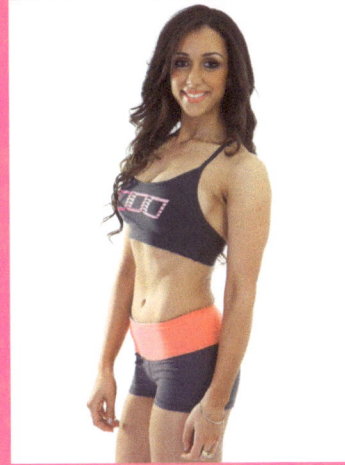

"When you live according to your highest values, you become inspired and awaken genius"

-John Demartini

SALLY'S STORY

Sally, 25, married, chiropractor

Now, I wake up daily with a picture in my mind of where I'm headed, and I just keep taking small steps to get where I want to go.

What an amazing ride Sally has had since she began her health journey at the age of 22!

Growing up, Sally was surrounded by a loving family. Although her family was close and caring, it wasn't a particularly healthy upbringing, with a diet that seemed to revolve around sugar. At times, Sally was actually served cake for dinner!

This diet resulted in a number of health problems for Sally. She suffered from neutropenia – a condition in which the type of white blood cell needed to help the body kill germs - especially bacteria – is missing. This left her more likely to get sick, and in her teenage years Sally had constant tonsillitis, middle ear infections, breathing issues, stomach aches and lethargy. She also had low bone density resulting in 14 bone fractures. Her calcium, iron and white blood cell levels were so low that doctors had to monitor her with blood tests every three months.

Sally rarely felt healthy; she just seemed to 'get through' her teenage years. This had an impact on her understanding of health, as she thought being healthy was simply not feeling sick. She didn't understand that being healthy meant feeling energised, vibrant and strong.

At 18, Sally began her studies in chiropractic care. With her heavy study load and weak health, she never really felt well. To boost her energy and mood, Sally started drinking coffee, and before long she found herself consuming up to 16 coffees a day. She began experiencing anxiety, heart palpitations, headaches and stomach upsets. She couldn't sleep at night and her day was a rollercoaster of feeling wired and then tired.

When she finally arrived at the end of her chiropractic studies at 22, Sally was 10kg overweight and constantly tired, sick and run down. Weeks later she received some tragic news. It was at this point she started to think about her health and the impact it was having on her life. Although she had studied nutrition and occasionally exercised, she began to realise that with her current lifestyle, she could not be a good role model to her future clients. So she decided things had to change.

Sally started by reflecting on her true values, to give her some clarity and purpose for her future goals. Her number one value, she discovered, was her health. This was an important discovery for Sally, as it allowed her to see that health had become the most crucial issue in her life. And she wanted to start feeling great, not just OK, so she began to visualise what she wanted to achieve and set specific goals based on these revelations.

With her values in mind, Sally created a vision board which helped to crystallise her goals. She cut out quotes and pictures of all the things she wanted to achieve and pasted them on her vision board, as well as on the fridge and the back of the bedroom door. She used these visual prompts as a subconscious reminder of where she was going and who she wanted to be. The vision board changed as Sally achieved each goal and looked to new aspirations.

Now that she had a direction, Sally wrote down all her goals, broke them into bite-sized pieces and got busy achieving them. She had the perfect starting point to take action as she had a visual reminder of where she was headed.

SALLY'S STATS: PHASE 1

	BEFORE	AFTER
Weight:	70kg	59kg
Dress Size:	12	10

Time from fat to fab: 20 weeks

Key to success: Creating a vision board, having a vision and setting tangible goals

SALLY'S STATS: PHASE 2
(Refining for photo cover competition)

	BEFORE	AFTER
Weight:	59kg	56kg
Dress Size:	10	8

Time from fat to fab: 12 weeks

Key to success: A finite goal date

Sally learnt about nutrition and gained the knowledge and tools to start making her vision and her health goals a reality. She completed a nutrition workshop, which gave her practical and simple techniques to implement the right changes for improved health and weight loss.

I asked Sally some questions about her journey

Tell us about the moment you decided to change your body and your health.
"I always knew I had to change my eating habits and start taking exercising seriously, but I thought I had plenty of time, as I was young and focused on my career. Health seemed like a distraction and I didn't want to face up to the reality of its importance in my life. Then a close friend died of a heart attack. Diet was a major part of the problem and he was only 24 years old. I was shocked and confused – how could this happen to someone so young? This was my wake up call. I realised I did *not* have plenty of time, so I began to turn my life around."

How did you begin your health-seeking journey?
"I had previously tried many things; boot camps, diets,

a lemon detox, naturopathy and more. Although each helped for a short while, I always put all the weight back on. I wanted to be someone whose good health was a reflection of their lifestyle. I seemed to be making small attempts, but never really lived as a healthy person, so I decided to change that. My gorgeous husband was, and still is, incredibly supportive. He encouraged me to keep trying different things and I eventually found something that was comfortable, a good fit for me and my values. It started with attending a workshop on healthy eating and something clicked. I had found what I was looking for".

How did you stay focused?

"I kept my vision in mind and always looked forward to where I wanted to be and what I wanted to achieve. Never looking back was the key to keeping me focused."

What challenges did you face?

"My family is of Middle Eastern descent and our culture looks at fuller-figured women as healthy. This made it difficult sometimes, as they would look at me and say "you look so fragile and thin – eat something". It felt like I was part of *My Big Fat Greek Wedding*! My family considers junk food and fried food as good. I understood it was OK to eat these foods sometimes, but we had different views on portion control! My family tends to indulge on a daily basis, or even with each meal, so I had to change my thinking and my habits to cater for my new way of eating."

How did you overcome these challenges?

"It is a work in progress. I knew my family acted from the kindness of their hearts. I tried to explain my point of view and what I was trying to achieve but parents will always parent you, no matter how old you are. So I accepted the situation and made small adjustments so things worked for me. I had my indulgent meal on the day I visited them and the rest of the time I planned healthy meals for the week."

How soon did you start to notice changes?

"I was surprised and very happy to discover that it was all a lot easier than I thought it was going to be. I changed my outlook on food and began changing my eating and exercise habits – one baby step at a time. Within a week I felt fantastic! This was a great motivational tool. With each small step, I felt healthier and stronger and my self-confidence was sky high."

And I believe you have a couple of secret weapons?

"My strategy was to learn from people who had already achieved similar goals. I thought about people I knew who had attained success with their health. I knew that it was easier to stand on the shoulders of giants and learn from their mistakes, rather than reinvent the wheel. I found some great role models and experts in the industry and did as they did, adapting their strategies to fit my lifestyle.

I also shared my goals and dreams with my husband and close friends. Although some of the goals were rather audacious, I believed the more people that knew my plans, the more likely I was to achieve them. It motivated me to work harder."

What advice do you have for a woman who wants to change her body?

"Go for it!! Every woman has her own insecurities, dramas and excuses, but the truth is that if you don't do anything about it, you'll always have the same issues with your body.

Write down your goals on paper so that they are out of your head and in the real world. Visualise achieving your goals and wake up every day thinking about what you can do that day to get closer to succeeding.

Surround yourself with like–minded people who are health conscious. Read good health resources, rather than magazines that make you feel terrible and give you the wrong message!

Be realistic with your steps – break them down to make them seem attainable. The easier it is, the more likely you will find success and be encouraged to keep going. Keep your vision in mind and don't let go of it, no matter what.

Getting healthy and lean was a lot easier in practice than I had imagined – and it will be for you, too. I am now a new person, both physically and mentally, and I have a wonderful relationship with food and my body. I now have the confidence to achieve whatever I set my heart and mind to."

Sally achieved remarkable results with the goals she had set for herself five months earlier. Step by step, she completely changed her lifestyle to a healthy one that she loved. She went from feeling like she'd run a marathon after running only a kilometre, to actually completing a real half marathon. And she looked and felt amazing. She was 59kg.

Over time, Sally's good lifestyle habits became automatic, so she actually found it easy to stay on track. She became a fine example to all her clients and was able to guide them with her first hand knowledge. With all these results under her belt, Sally was itching for a new challenge. She decided to enter a magazine front cover competition and get the body of a goddess at the same time!

So began 12 weeks of goal setting and achieving. The first step was to create a weekly eating plan and exercise program. Sally listed every food she enjoyed that was healthy and stocked her cupboards and fridge. Then she started eating only these foods. Her sense of purpose was strong and she was resolved to eat clean, healthy food for a healthy body and mind.

"I now have no problem sticking to set targets, and I knew where I was heading. As I refined my food even further I felt even better, which just encouraged me

to continue eating this way. Every time I made an improvement, I noticed a positive and exhilarating flow on effect. This has made it a lot easier to maintain."

Get Ready to Kick Goals

"Obstacles are what you see when you take your eyes off your goals"
Brian Tracy

Whether it is the desire for more money, improved relationships, a successful career or a healthy, fit body, we all have goals. Many goals are just vague ideas about things we want to change. Our goals are often the opposite of the things we complain about on a daily basis! These goals are fuzzy and unclear; they are concepts rather than tangible targets.

The key to success with goals is to clarify exactly what you want to achieve and lay out an action plan to get there. In order to become clear about exactly what you want to achieve, begin by defining and outlining what is important to you. This will give you a clear picture of where you are and what you need to do next.

Values

Values are a set of principles and beliefs that are of ultimate importance to each of us. They are the essence of what drives you towards taking particular actions.

Your values reflect what you do and who you are today

Knowing what your values are will help you determine what your focus is, and from there, where you want to be. If you truly want to change your health and your body, you need to work out how health can become your number one value.

Firstly, start by considering your TRUE core values - not those you think you should live by according to society's influences. Is success, family, health, wealth, happiness, contentment, self-esteem or perhaps fame important to you?

Write down your top 5 values

_____

_____

_____

_____

_____

Tip

Ask yourself, "What do I get excited about and put most of your energy towards?" Consider your answers in relation to **what you are actually doing right now** in your life. If you need prompting, see the list below.

List of Values

Abundance	Determination	Power	Satisfying others
Acceptance	Devotion	Practicality	Security
Accomplishment	Discipline	Problem Solving	Service (to others)
Accountability	Efficiency	Knowledge	Significance
Adventure	Empathy	Leadership	Simplicity
Balance	Energy	Love or Romance	Skill
Beauty	Equality	Mastery	Spirituality
Brilliance	Excellence	Meaning	Stability
Calmness	Fairness	Merit	Status
Challenge	Faith	Motivation	Strength
Change	Family	Openness	Success (achievement)
Charity	Fitness	Orderliness	Synergy
Commitment	Freedom	Passion	Teamwork
Communication	Friendship	Patience	Tolerance
Community	Fun	Perfection	Tradition
Competence	Good will	Persistence	Tranquillity
Competition	Gratitude	Personal Growth	Trust
Concern for others	Happiness	Pleasure	Truth
Contentment	Harmony	Positive attitude	Unity
Improvement	Health (physical)	Progress	Variety
Cooperation	Health (emotional)	Prosperity	Vision
Coordination	Honesty	Punctuality	Vitality
Courtesy	Honour	Quality of work	Wealth
Creativity	Independence	Respect	Wellbeing
Decisiveness	Integrity	Responsiveness	Wisdom

Adapted from: © FBP and Associates – 2006 Commonly Held Values

If you have listed values that seem to have no relevance to your health, think again. You can entwine them to ensure your health rates highly on your list.

If family is the most important priority, for example, keeping fit enough to play with your kids could be one way of getting fitness into your top five values. If you listed success, satisfaction, confidence or happiness, all of these can relate to health. That is, if you achieve great health, all of these values are amplified. If how you look or how you feel is very important to you, a good diet is vital. Even values such as pleasure, achievement and

altruism can relate to your health. For example, you can take pleasure in exercising and eating well, attaining an improved state of health, or seek altruism by helping others improve their health too.

Once you have a solid list of values, you can create goals that accurately reflect what is important to you. If you are passionate about what you are trying to achieve, you will have a much greater chance of success.

Goal Attack

"Committing your goals to paper increases the likelihood of your achieving them by one thousand percent"
Brian Tracy

Setting SMART goals

The SMARTer goal setting technique is a simple method which allows you to make your goals real for you. SMART is an acronym for goals that are Specific, Measurable, Action-based, Realistic and Time-based.

Specific - A specific goal maximises your chance of success as it focuses your attention and energy on what you need to do to achieve your goals.

Change:	To specific:
I want to lose weight	I will lose one dress size and run three times a week for 20 minutes

Measurable - If you can't measure your goal, how will you know that you have reached it? When you measure your progress, you stay on track and experience the exhilaration of achievement, which in turn spurs you on to achieve even more! Make sure you have numbers and dates set.

Change:	To measurable:
I will start exercising and eat better	I will walk 3km every day and re-stock my pantry with healthy food by Friday

Action-based - Having clear action steps to achieve your goals is critical to goal setting success. Ask yourself: "What steps do I need to take and what resources do I need to achieve my goals?"

Goal:	Steps: How am I going to achieve this?
I want to lose 5kg in four months	I will replace my morning biscuit with a healthy snack I will take a healthy lunch to work I will eat fish three times a week and no takeaway food I will get up at 6.30am and walk or jog for 20 minutes

Realistic - Setting realistic goals does not necessarily mean the goals are easy, but they must be achievable. If you have never run 1km, there is little use in setting a goal to run a marathon in four weeks. Likewise, if you hate Brussels sprouts and zucchini, don't vow to include them in your meals. By setting unrealistic goals you are setting yourself up for failure, which does not help your self-confidence or your ability to achieve other goals.

Instead, set a goal that you can imagine yourself carrying through with. Experiencing success with these goals will encourage you to aim higher.

Goal:	Steps: How am I going to achieve this?
Eat less chocolate	I will have two squares the nights I feel like it

Time-based - When you set a deadline to achieve your goals, you create a sense of urgency to take action! Whether your time frame is today, tomorrow or in five years, clearly define an end date to make your goals a priority. Include plenty of short-term goals so that you experience regular success.

Getting SMARTer

I like to set **SMARTer** goals, not just SMART. Consider whether you are setting goals that are:

Energising - Are your SMART goals energetic and do they evoke emotion? You must be passionate about achieving your goals to be motivated to keep on track.

Reviewed - Research on athletes and successful business people shows that regularly reviewing your goals maximises your chances of success. Over time, your priorities and circumstances will change. You might also find there are obstacles and difficulties to achieving your goals, so a slight change in direction may be needed. If you can, enlist the help of a mentor or friend who can monitor your goals weekly or fortnightly for you.

Goal:	Steps: How am I going to achieve this?
Eat healthy food	In one week I will have a pantry full of healthy food
	In one week I will have weekly meals planned for the following week
	In three weeks I will have cooked 20 healthy recipes I enjoy eating and will rotate them for two months
Replace all takeaway foods	In two weeks I will have five alternatives to takeaway

Goal Setting Tips

1. Frame your goals in positive statements

2. Write your goals down and keep them where you can see them

3. Pick goals that are important to you and are in line with your vision

4. Make a public commitment to your goal – tell everyone!

5. Reward yourself when you reach a goal

Your Goal Setting Toolbox

"Deep inside, you have a desire to fulfil that which is most important in your life"
Dr John Demartini

Once you have established what is truly important to you in your life, you can explore and implement some tools to really bring your goals to life. These strategies will enable you to lay out your dreams with clarity and purpose. Find a technique that calls out to you and allows you to specifically plan forward for your success.

Vision Board

A vision board is a collage of images and words depicting what you want to bring into your life. It helps to plant a picture in your subconscious mind, reminding you what you want and allowing you to see where you are headed. Vision boards are an effective planning tool to set you on the path towards your desired future. There are many reports of people attracting their goals into their lives once they have created them on a vision board.

I have a vision board in my wardrobe which helps keep me focused. I have photos of healthy food, fit people, scenes of holidays, sleeping soundly and meaningful words. The picture of a fit runner reminds me of the importance of running in my life.

My Vision Board

To create your own vision board, start with a large piece of cardboard. Select pictures and words from magazines and websites to create a collage of images that represent you and what you want. Paste pictures or write words that fill you with passion and positive emotions. Include pictures and photos of the body you want and healthy foods you like to eat.

Put copies of your vision board in your heaviest traffic zones – on the wall where you get dressed, in the bathroom, on the fridge, at your desk, in your wallet, as a screensaver. The more you see it, the sooner your subconscious will believe it to be real and help to guide you in that direction.

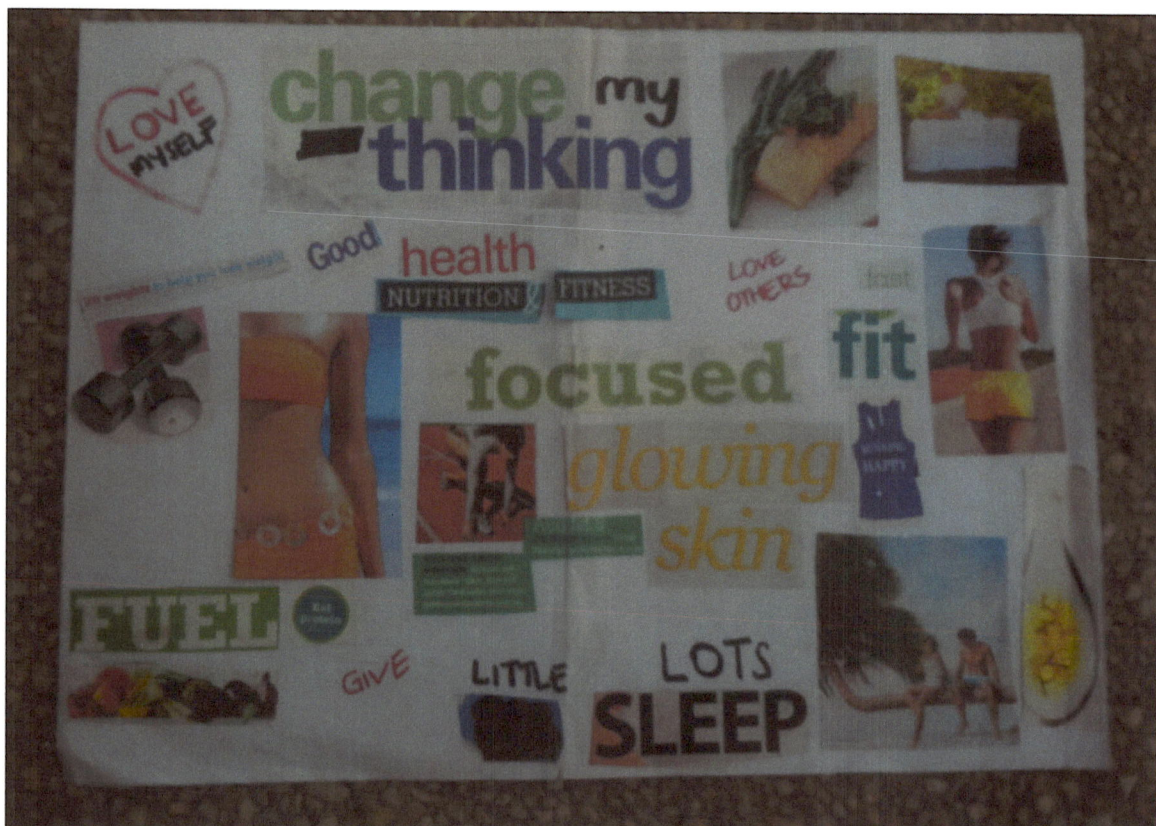

Visualisation

"Ordinary people believe only in the possible. Extraordinary people visualise not what is possible or probable, but rather what is impossible. And by visualising the impossible, they begin to see it as possible"
Cherie Carter-Scott

Visualisation is the technique of using your imagination to visualise specific events happening in your life. By imagining your goal over and over, your mind begins to see it as reality. Use all your senses when you visualise – what do you see, smell, feel and hear when you imagine having achieved your goal?

The mind is an amazing tool. If you imagine taking a bite out of a juicy lemon and really make it seem real, you will salivate as though you had really taken a bite. If you vividly imagine yourself riding a bike, your heart rate will increase as if you really were exercising.

Visualisation is a powerful way to bring about what you want in your life. All the ladies in these stories imagined themselves as they wanted to be. Just like the athlete imagines herself winning her race, you can visualise yourself getting where you want to go.

The most effective time to visualise is when you are falling asleep or waking up. Start practising visualising what you want to see come true when you go to bed and when you wake in the morning. Each time you practise it becomes easier, and the vision becomes clearer. Soon it will become your reality.

Mind Map

"A mind map is a thinking tool that reflects what goes on inside your head"
Tony Buzan, creator of the mind mapping technique

Drawing and writing your dreams and goals in a creative way releases your thoughts from your mind and on to paper. The process de-clutters any confused thoughts and may even reveal thoughts you weren't conscious of. It can help bring clarity to the process of goal setting and increase your understanding of what you really want.

A few years ago I was completely lost and stagnant in my career. It was a confusing time, and I had no idea what direction I wanted to take. There were so many ideas swimming around in my head, but I was stuck without answers for many months. A friend suggested I create a mind map and the result was fantastic. As soon as all the thoughts were out of my head, my mind was clear and I was ready for action. It is amazing how it suddenly became so crystal clear to me what I wanted to do.

Within weeks I started running healthy eating workshops as well as cooking classes. My business grew and my message reached a much greater audience. My health goals became clearer and I mapped out what I wanted to achieve. The mind map revealed desires and ideas I never knew existed and enabled me to take action and pursue my dreams with conviction.

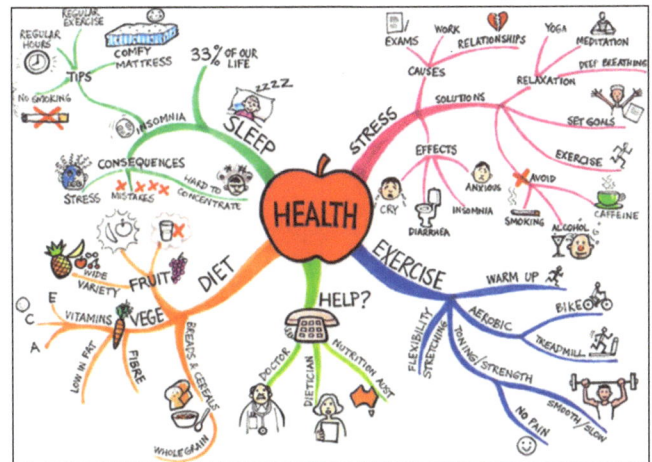

Source: www.learningfundamentals.com.au/wp-content/uploads/health-map.jpg

You can create your own mind map focused on your health. Start with a blank piece of paper and draw a colourful picture in the centre of the page. In the picture, write 'HEALTH'. Then draw wavy branches away from the picture. The lines will look like the branches of a tree. On these lines, write out whatever comes to mind in relation to your health – in one word. Let your mind wander and let the words come naturally from within. Give yourself permission to write down whatever surfaces.

Just as our thoughts tend to go off in branches as one idea leads to another, you may find you'd like to add smaller branches to the original lines. Go with it, as the smaller branches can hold extra ideas that you would like to consider. One project you would like to take on could lead in many different possible directions, so this is where you can record all the possibilities.

As you reflect back on your mind map, you will become clearer on which branch is the one you wish to follow first. The words along that branch can become the foundation for developing your plan of action.

Storyboarding

Storyboarding is simply creating a story on boards – a graphic organiser. Screenwriters use this technique to show the direction of a movie or screenplay from beginning to end. It allows the team to get a clear picture of where each scene is headed.

You can use this planning strategy to provide clarity and direction for your goals. It enables you to create consecutive steps towards your desired outcome. I used the storyboard technique to get the words to start flowing for this book. It gave me a clear framework to establish format and direction.

To create your own storyboard, write out what you want to achieve in a single sentence, for example: 'To be fit and strong'. What is the first thing you need to do to bring your dream to fruition? Then write the second and third step. Look for themes or patterns that appear to provide you with direction. The pages might look something like this:

RESEARCH	**GET READY**	**MEASURE & REFINE**	**SET GOALS AND PLAN**
1. Join the gym 2. Start playing tennis 3. Recruit support Local Gym: Ph: 23456788 Tennis Club: Ph: 12345678 Call Jane	1. Buy gear - running shoes, skipping rope 2. Set up area for home exercise 3. Set alarm 4. Get gym program from trainer 5. Choose gym classes	1 month – review goals 3 months – review goals and set new weekly and monthly goals	1. Put my goal end dates for the week and month into my diary 2. Register for fun run

Facing Your Fears

Once we have decided to make change in our lives, the unfortunate reality is that most of us will come up against obstacles or fears that make change more difficult.

According to human behavioural specialists, there are two major fears, or obstacles, to achieving goals. Can you relate to either of these fears?

1. Do you think others have something you don't that makes their success come easier? Do you think others can succeed because they are luckier, richer or more intelligent than you? The reality is that everyone has their own challenges and their own skills. Comparing yourself to others won't help you or them. It's not worth the effort!

2. Do you have a fear of failure? This fear is the concern that change could bring about more pain than pleasure. Getting it wrong may be disastrous, so it may seem easier to do nothing at all. Take a tip from babies: despite failing again and again, they never stop trying to walk. And slowly but surely, they reach their goal. Failure is simply feedback advising you to refine your approach. Mistakes are an opportunity to achieve great things.

Once you clear your mind of obstacles and fears, you will experience more clarity with your goals and find it easier to move towards them.

"Mistakes are the perfect opportunity to learn and achieve great things"

Action

Mind...

On a large piece of paper, start writing down your goals in all facets of your life. Let your imagination run wild and write down everything – big dreams, small goals and hopes for the future. Goals in all areas of your life are interconnected and have an impact on each other. For example:

Health	Family	Career	Financial	Social	Mental	Spiritual
Run 10km	Weekly activity	Own business	Earn $x this year	Call a friend daily	Contentment	Charity work
Eat healthy food	Play together	Study	Save 10%	Weekly outing	Achievement	Meditation
Feel energised	Weekends away	Work with 15 clients a week	Buy an investment property		Self Development	
Lose 5kg						

Now add more detail to your HEALTH goals. Use other strategies – visualisation, a mind map and storyboard, as described above, to help clarify your goals and direction.

Body & Food...

Make sure you have listed all your food and exercise goals. Break each health goal into bite-size pieces. For example, to run 10km, join a running group, enlist the help of an expert, buy new running shoes, sign up for a fun run. To eat healthy food, list the steps – fill the pantry and fridge with healthy food, plan out meals ahead, change what you eat for breakfast and enrol in some healthy cooking classes.

For example:

Health Goals	Goal Break Down – Action Steps
Run 10km	Enter a fun run, join a running group, find a running coach or friend to train with
Eat healthy food	Prepare menu for the week using healthy, tasty meals Go shopping for the ingredients as well as healthy snacks
Feel energised and healthy	Eat regularly, eat fresh foods and start exercising a few times a week
Join a sporting group	Search the internet for local clubs and visit those ones that seem suitable
Cook new healthy recipes	Search key phrases and cooking websites, print recipes and start cooking today
Lose 5kg	Eat small meals regularly, eat more protein and vegetables, don't overeat, take measurements and photos

Write down every single step you need to take. Sometimes the most difficult task is to take the first step – then things get easier once you get the ball rolling. Always assume there will be obstacles, because there always will be, so list potential solutions to any foreseeable issues. For example, sickness, holidays and work demands – we all have them!

TIP: Choose visuals of these goals for your vision board, or make a list of goals to put up around the house. Remember to review your goals regularly.

Eating Your Way to Great Health

Before: 100kg

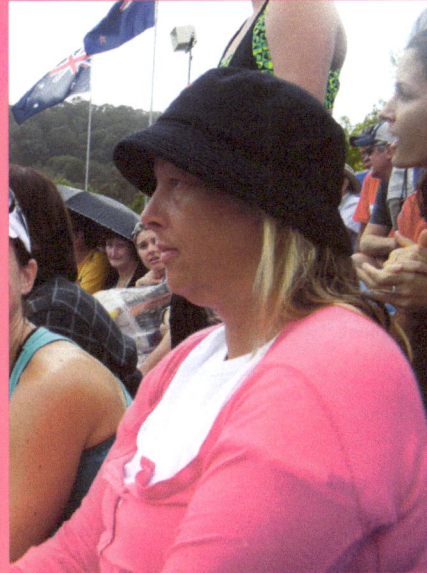

"Now I sit down to eat and take my time. It made a huge difference to how I felt as well as to my waistline!"

LIZ'S STORY

Liz, 44, mother of three, personal trainer and fitness instructor

Liz spent many years on the dieting rollercoaster. She would lose a little, gain a lot, try new diets and lose weight through stress. She had a lot of challenges throughout the years as a working mother of three. At 35, she found herself weighing 85kg, at 39 hit 90kg and by age 43 at 100kg, she really started to despair. At that time, she also had some serious personal problems to deal with and she was using food for comfort and as a stress release. Her self-esteem was at an all-time low and she was in a place she no longer wanted to be. She 'disappeared', becoming someone she didn't know or particularly like. And then on one particular day, she saw a photo of herself and decided that was the day things had to change.

After: 75kg

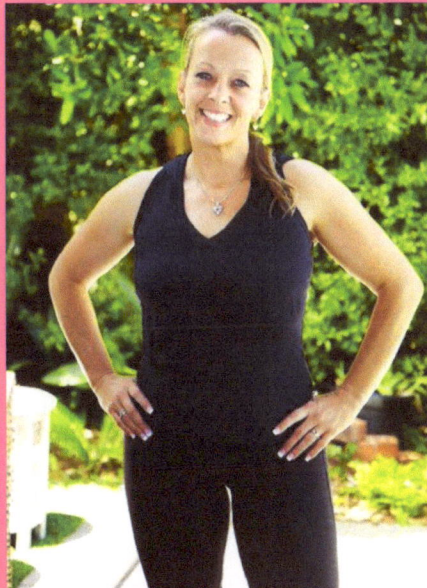

Liz wasn't sure where to begin, but she thought that writing things on paper would give her some clarity and direction. She starting writing down the reasons why she wanted to get healthy and lose the weight. She couldn't believe how quickly she filled the pages and ended up with 100 reasons. This was the trigger that really got her inspired to change. She discovered the number one reason she wanted to change was the need to give to herself.

Liz started by allocating one full hour every day to exercising – whether it was alone or with her husband. She found his support and his love of fitness to be motivating in the times she needed a little encouragement. Only a few weeks later, Liz had improved her fitness and was feeling better. She found the time out to be nurturing and therapeutic.

After several months, Liz was enjoying her new-found fitness and progressing well with her weight loss until she hit a plateau with 15kg to go. She still wasn't feeling truly healthy.

Even though she was now fit and eating a little better, she knew she needed to train smarter and completely change her eating habits if she wanted to lose the rest of the weight. Liz came to see me and we looked at how she was eating.

Liz's food habits were almost the opposite of how they needed to be! She was eating a small breakfast, snacking through the day and then eating a large dinner at night. Her lack of food during the day meant she was starving by dinner time and would overeat. She was so busy during the day that she would quickly grab whatever was available and eat it fast, and her hunger at night meant she also ate her dinner too quickly.

She was continually tired and bloated, with little energy when she most needed it. During the day, she ate lollies and drank coffee to lift her energy, but she would soon come crashing down and then repeat this cycle.

We constructed an eating strategy to address her energy levels and fat loss goals. This included

LIZ'S STATS		
	BEFORE	**AFTER**
Weight	100kg	75kg
Dress Size	18-20	14
Time from fat to fab: 6 months		
Key to success: Being prepared for the day		

structured preparation time for her meals and an education in how to eat. With her preparation and plans in hand, Liz's good eating habits *became* a habit. She carried her food supplies with her each day and cooked extra at night for the following day. She started to find the extra fat was rapidly disappearing.

Liz also decided to become a personal trainer as she wanted to live the life of fitness. She completed her personal training course and when qualified, secured a job as a gym instructor at her fitness centre and began training clients of her own. Liz had begun living her life as a fit and healthy personal trainer – and she loved it.

Liz went on to achieve all her goals within six months. At 45, she had become a strong, lean happy woman – and a brilliant role model for all her clients. Women were inspired by her energy and strength – she really was a formidable force! Liz learnt she could achieve anything, and soon set her sights on triathlons and a body sculpting competition.

NOTE: Find out in Step 5 how she trained less for better weight loss results…

I asked Liz some questions about her journey

When was your life-changing moment?
"The crunch came when I saw photos of myself on holidays…. it shocked the hell out of me and I thought: "How have I done this to myself? So I started listing the reasons why I wanted to 'give up' being so unhealthy. I realised if I didn't do anything about it, I would face some serious health problems in the near future. I already had severe knee pain and I knew it was due

to my weight. It had become impossible to ride a bike without excruciating pain. All these factors made me realise it was time to change."

What has been your most difficult challenge in your quest for the body you wanted?

"The most difficult challenge I faced was believing in myself enough to start the recovery process. I avoided dealing with it for a long time by keeping busy, and was using food as a source of comfort. So ending this cycle was very difficult. I had forgotten to be me, I had taken on the role of wife and mother and, although I loved my family, I lost myself in the process."

How did you begin?

"I began by getting fit again and changing my diet a little. It really got the ball rolling and I lost quite a bit of weight. But when I plateaued with my progress, I knew I had to really look at my eating habits. As I was inspired by what I had already achieved, I was motivated to do whatever I needed to do to keep progressing."

Did changing HOW you ate make a difference?

"Changing how I ate was the solution for me. I learnt that I was not eating enough at each meal or snack and I was not eating frequently enough. I started eating more slowly and noticed I was really enjoying my food again! Slowing down also stopped me from eating until I was too full, which was a new experience for me.

The quality of food I had been eating was OK, but I had made no real progress until I changed my way of eating. I am now mindful of how I eat; I always sit down now and take my time – it made a huge difference to how I felt and to my waistline!"

How did your preparation help you to achieve your dreams?

"I had my eating patterns professionally reviewed – how and when, as well as what I was eating. I had always thought I ate pretty well, but discovered I had to learn to get prepared and to eat more regularly. I learnt how to change my daily habits and it made a huge difference.

I started carrying around snacks and meals during the day, and when it came to working at night I was energised, rather than tired. Being organised kept me on track – I felt so great I couldn't give it up! I combined this with weight training and bike riding.... the results were fantastic."

What challenges did you face along the way? How did you overcome them?

"The days I was not prepared or organised with my food were the days I ate poorly. On those occasions, I was taking the easy way out and grabbing anything available, rather than considering what was the most suitable option to fuel myself. So I was over-hungry and making unhealthy food choices by the end of the day, as I was starving! It didn't take me long to realise this was not helping me reach my goals. So I made sure I always had plenty of healthy food options on hand and it soon became easy to eat well every day.

Icy winter mornings were a challenge, so I found a partner to train with. This kept me accountable and made training a lot more fun. We motivated each other and shared what we had learnt. I highly recommend you do this if you will be exercising early in the day.

Finally, alcohol was challenging my quest for great health and fat loss. Socialising took on a whole new look. Soda water and fresh lime became my drink of choice most of the time, and although I missed the champagne initially, I soon got used to it. Now I just have a glass of champagne if I really feel like it, as opposed to for the sake of it! And I never have to face hangovers, eat junk food or feel exhausted for the entire following day as I used to most weekends. I felt so great once I was showing my body a little more respect, and I had the energy to eat well and exercise on the weekends."

How did you stay on track?

"*How you feel* is the best motivator. When I cleaned up my diet, I felt brilliant and was full of energy. If I didn't eat well I felt terrible. It was a simple solution to keep me on track. I loved how I felt every day, as opposed to just getting through each day feeling tired and irritable. My snack pack became my new best friend. I started to see the weight fall off, which was a great source of motivation. Also, my knee pain disappeared, so I could do any activity I wanted – which helped me stay fit.

I also kept a check on my progress. Measurements were effective for me; it was motivating to see the changes taking place on a chart as well as in the mirror. I also began receiving compliments, which was very inspiring.

I think most mums put their family before themselves; it is part of the unconditional love that comes with the job, but we have to remember, it all starts with ourselves. By allowing *me* to be my focus for the first time in a very long time, I was able to slowly regain my sense of self, and in time, be proud of me. I was also lucky to have had the support and love of my husband and kids, as without them I would have struggled.

When I decided to follow my dream of working in the fitness industry, I was able to relate to others who were starting out in the position I had been in. It was very rewarding and being a role model to others also keeps me on track.

I have maintained my weight for over twelve months and have succeeded at achieving each new goal I have set for myself. My next goal is to compete in the upcoming triathlon season..... I can't wait!"

What advice do you have for a woman who wants to change her body?

"Write down 100 reasons why you want to change your health and your life; it's a great incentive to get you started. Keep reminding yourself of where you are headed, and when you're finding it tough. Keep in mind that thousands of women have been on this journey too, and they have succeeded. Talk to friends and like-minded women and seek support and reassurance. Don't be afraid to ask for help; we all have - it will keep you focused on your dreams."

How to Use Food to Reach Your Goals

"Before anything else, preparation is the key to success"
Alexander Graham Bell

Many people focus only on *what* to eat, yet if you learn *how* and *when* to eat you will discover how much you really need to consume in order to lose the fat and feel brilliant.

Our body is a finely tuned machine which knows when it needs to be fuelled. This is the often overlooked signal of HUNGER. Our body is designed to tell us when to eat by releasing a hormone which sends our brain a hunger signal. We have an inbuilt homeostatic mechanism, which attempts to maintain a static weight. If this hunger signal is repeatedly ignored, our body will eventually respond by decreasing our metabolic rate and our body will become very effective at storing fat.

In order to reach our desired weight or body fat level, we must listen to our bodies as well as engage in 'mindful eating'. For some people, this means eating more frequently, others need to eat less at each meal, whilst some may simply need to eat more good quality foods.

Mindful Eating

Mindfulness is simply the moment-by-moment awareness of life. But it's not always easy to be present in the moment. We get caught up in our own thoughts, what we need to do next or what we have done in the past, and the present moment gets little attention. This is true of how we eat too. Some of us eat meal after meal, snack after snack, barely aware of what we're eating and how much we're consuming.

Mindfulness is a return to paying attention to life. When we pay attention to our food – really pay attention – we begin to notice all sorts of wonderful aspects to the food we eat, and we also become aware of when to eat and how much we're putting into our bodies.

Eat when you are hungry

It's time to eat when the hunger signal alerts you. It seems obvious, but many of us eat when we are not hungry. We eat for many reasons, including boredom, emotions, routine, in social settings or when we are over-hungry. This is a good recipe for excessive intake and making less nutritious choices.

Fuel your body when it asks, as it is telling you it needs food and can use the energy source now. Your body will begin to adapt and you will start to lose the fat and surge with energy.

In order to eat at the right time, it is imperative that you are prepared. If you are surrounded by healthy foods you can eat well when your body sends you the signal that it's time to eat. It will be easier to make healthy choices with foods that keep you satisfied for longer.

What if you are one of those people who rarely feel hungry? This is usually the result of years of ignoring the hunger signals, so it's time to switch them back on. This begins with how you feel when you wake up in the morning. If you do not feel hungry in the morning, your metabolism is probably sluggish and you will need to re-train your body.

Your goal is to wake up feeling hungry, so if you don't feel like food, have something small, such as a piece of fruit or a smoothie. You will find that within a few days, you are feeling hungrier in the morning. Don't be frightened by this, it doesn't mean you will want to eat all day. The opposite is true; if you start your day by fuelling your body when it needs it, your hunger will be much less by the end of the day. You won't be starving by dinner time, so you will avoid over-eating or choosing less healthy foods. Your body certainly doesn't need much fuel in the evening as it winds down for the day, when you are most likely sitting on the couch!

If you are truly hungry before bed, have a serve of protein

This ensures you have enough protein to get you through the night as your body repairs, rebuilds and rejuvenates!

Are you really hungry?

Real hunger is a calm desire for food which gradually develops and should be attended to while the signal is mild.

Water hunger has the same characteristics, so it may be mistaken for real hunger. To avoid this, drink water regularly, ideally around 200ml per hour.

Blood sugar hunger strikes when your blood sugar levels drop too low (hypoglycaemia). This creates sugar cravings and a fast, powerful desire to eat. It is a strong form of hunger, as the body must act quickly to ensure enough sugar is provided to fuel the brain.

Addictive substance hunger comes from the removal of an addictive food such as sugar or wheat. It is a subtle form of hunger that only lasts a short amount of time. It can be difficult to let go of, as it reinforces the belief that the addictive food is giving you something you need.

Nutrient imbalance hunger occurs when you consume a meal with an incorrect ratio of protein, carbohydrates and fat. It usually creates the strongest feeling of hunger, which also leaves you with an empty feeling. It is a biochemical imbalance which creates sugar cravings, moodiness and a strong desire to eat again between 15 minutes and 3 hours after a meal.

Emotional hunger is psychological rather than physical, and manifests itself in cravings which have an almost instantaneous onset. Particular thoughts provide the triggers to eat.

Eat regularly

Eating smaller meals more frequently will help burn more calories as it will boost your metabolism. Aim to eat every 3 to 4 hours, with a pattern something like this:

7am: breakfast	10am: snack
12.30pm: lunch	3pm: snack
7pm: small dinner	9pm: snack if hungry

This is a general guide only. Try not to eat by the clock. Use your hunger signals – your body knows when it's hungry! If you are hungry at 11.30, have your lunch then, or have half your lunch and the other half when you are next hungry. Eating strictly by the clock may encourage you to eat when you are not really hungry. If you have your food prepared, you can simply eat when your body needs it.

One of the common times we get hungry is around 3-4pm. Having a snack around this time is vital to:

1) keep you fuelled and your insulin levels stable, allowing your body to release fat stores to be used as your energy source
2) ensure you get enough protein
3) increase your metabolism
4) stop you from overeating at dinner time and after dinner and storing extra calories
5) prevent you from getting over-hungry and stopping for takeaway on the way home!

Sit down, eat slowly and enjoy your food

- Always eat when you are sitting down. Choose one or two areas at home and at work and only eat in those places, rather than while standing over the sink or walking around. You will enjoy your meal more, which is what it's all about! Becoming truly aware of what you are eating is a wonderful experience.

- Take a deep breath before you begin eating. This will help you to stop and think about what you are about to eat and how you will eat it. Look at your food and take the time to enjoy it.

- Digestion begins in your mouth; there are actually more digestive enzymes in the mouth than in the stomach. Chew slowly to break down your food and digest it more efficiently. This prevents inflammation and bloating and allows the body to be in a better state to lose the weight and feel great.

Many people starve themselves while thinking about food all day, and then proceed to gobble their evening meal in five minutes. Eating slowly means the signal that you are full will reach the brain before you overeat. In a study published in the *Journal of the American Dietetics Association* in 2008, subjects reported feeling fuller when they ate slowly. They also ended up consuming about 10% fewer calories when they ate at a slow pace rather than rushing. Another study published in the *British Medical Journal in 2008,* found that eating quickly, and eating until feeling full, tripled subjects' risk of being overweight.

If you stop to think about what you are eating and eat in the moment, you will enjoy it more, eat more slowly, digest it better and not overeat!

Stop when you are satisfied – do not overeat

Many of us eat too much in one sitting and barely notice it. If you stopped overeating in a sitting by as little as a large handful of chips or ½ a muesli slice, you would lose 5kg in a year! Now that's worth thinking about. Plus, who really likes the feeling of eating too much? It's an uncomfortable feeling, which also promotes weight gain.

Becoming aware helps you eat the right amount

The more aware of how you are eating, the less likely you will be to overeat. Think about a time you ate too much. How did you feel? Bloated, uncomfortable, perhaps miserable for doing it? It's not something you want in your life! You don't *need* to overeat – you can eat again the next time you feel hungry!

Keep this powerful thought in your mind: "I can eat whenever I am hungry." This will prevent you from feeling any uneasiness or panic about not being 'allowed' to eat what you need. Try pausing in the middle of your meal for a couple of minutes. Estimate how much more food it will take to fill you comfortably. This really raises your awareness of how much you are eating. It does not mean you need to eat a low calorie diet, just eat when you are hungry and stop when you are satisfied.

When you eat with the intention of feeling better after a meal, you are less likely to keep eating until the plate is empty

It is a great feeling to be satisfied but not excessively full. Especially at dinner time, always eat a little less than you think you need. If you have eaten regularly throughout the day you will not feel like eating a large dinner, as you have already met the day's energy requirements.

Move your plate away or get up from the table as soon as you feel satisfied. The desire to keep eating will pass quickly. Just remember that you can eat again whenever you are hungry. Once you stop the habit of overeating, you will never want to do it again. It is actually an easy habit to break, as you will remember that uncomfortable feeling and never want to repeat it.

Allow yourself to eat what you want – the 80/20 rule

Having a list of foods that you are not allowed to eat only makes you desire them more. The forbidden is always very desirable! It's amazing how the desire for less healthy foods diminishes significantly when you

know you *can* have them. Knowing that a food is not forbidden means that if you do eat unhealthy foods, you will usually consume a lot less volume a lot less often.

If you eat really well at least 80% of the time, you have some leeway to eat less nutritious foods the other 20% of the time and still get results. Obviously the better your diet, the better the results will be, but remove the concept of forbidden foods from your life – it will help keep you on track. Having a piece of cake or a burger occasionally does not make you fat. What does make you fat is eating at the wrong times, not eating enough, overeating and not eating satisfying foods.

Shopping for Success

Before you launch into your new eating plan, it is important to have the right foods around you. If there is one golden rule with preparation, this is it. Surround yourself with healthy foods at home, in the office, in the car and wherever else you regularly spend time. If it's in reach, you will automatically choose healthy foods most of the time. The effort spent on being prepared is vital to your ongoing success – and it is also much easier than having to go out of your way to look for good food every few hours.

Clear out your pantry and fridge

Start by removing all items you know are unhealthy from your home and office. Having these foods around will only prolong reaching your goals. You may be reluctant to waste food, so give it to the needy or an appreciative recipient. If the chips and chocolate are not in the cupboard, you will rarely desire them, and if you really want them, you will make the effort to go to the shop to get them.

If you work in an office, store non-perishables in the kitchen cupboard and take fresh food on Mondays to keep in the fridge or freezer. Stock the office as if it was your second home.

Keep healthy non-perishables in a carry bag in your car for emergencies.

Decide Where to Shop

Create a list of quality shops you can visit regularly to do your shopping. It may help if your shopping day is the same each week to establish a routine and stay on track.

Consider the following:

a) Farmers' market or local organic producers – fruit, vegetables

Local organic fruit and vegetable growers often home deliver. The produce they grow can be cheaper than supermarket produce, and it ensures you get enough fruit and vegetables on a weekly basis. It's also a lot easier, fresher and tastier – so start investigating!

TIP: Colourful fruits and vegetables are highly nutritious and brilliant for fat loss, so eat lots! Pick up a fruit and vegetable seasonal guide from your local fruit shop or producer.

b) Butcher – meat supplies and healthy quick meals

A good butcher will source high quality produce. They may offer chemical-free choices and some prepare their own ham and roast turkey. You might even find ready-made meals such as soups, burgers and meat sauces. This is a much healthier option than the artificially produced products in the supermarket and tastes so much better.

c) Deli - cold meats, olives, seafood, cooked chicken

If you need to buy seafood at the deli, check that the seafood is fresh. Ask to smell the produce – there should be no 'fishy' odour.

Research shows that a high consumption of processed meat increases your risk of stomach and pancreatic cancer, so keep your intake to less than 50g per day (a couple of slices). To reduce the risk, select the most natural, additive-free products available. It's a tough ask, but if you want to avoid chemicals and artificial ingredients, buy organic deli meats. As organic products don't contain preservatives, store them well and consume them within one or two days.

d) Supermarket

Hit the supermarket with your eyes wide open.

Discover the health food section, different vegetables, and peruse the deli and the canned goods aisle for healthy options.

Stock up on your staples, ensuring the ingredients list is as short and as natural as possible, and choose organic, if possible. You can buy organic cans, pastas, cereals and rice. Browse the health food aisle, but make sure you read the labels, as plenty of foods in this area are *not* healthy. You can also investigate healthy convenient food options, such as cold soups and more natural, ready-to-go meals.

e) Health food store

Browse your local health food stores for other specialty items not in the supermarket. They will have a wider range of healthy items and some good snack food options. Hunt down the most qualified staff and ask them as many questions as you can to improve your knowledge.

Plan your meals

Planning your menu will be invaluable. It does require some forethought, but ultimately it will make things much easier to manage. It will help you establish your shopping list and relieve you of having to make food decisions every day of the week.

If you find yourself pressed for time or the head space to cook a healthy meal each night, cook in batches. When you do have time to cook a meal, make double the amount, and freeze or keep leftovers fresh in the fridge. It takes about the same amount of time to cook twice as much, and you will have meals ready for nights you don't have time to cook.

If it's more your style to plan a day ahead, cook just a little extra dinner to cater for breakfast, lunch or dinner the next day. An extra chicken fillet and roast sweet potato is perfect to add to a warm salad for lunch.

We all know how valuable our spare time is, so keep life simple by thinking ahead a little. A small amount of planning saves you a lot of time, thought and possibly money if it prevents you from hitting the drive-through or calling for takeaway.

Create a shopping list

Use the sample shopping list to give you ideas. Once you are settled into your new eating routine you can expand on this list to include as much variety as you like. You may be surprised by the wide range of healthy foods available for your new menu!

Pantry

Beans and legumes (dried or canned) - lentils, cannellini, borlotti, red kidney, butter, black, black-eyed, lima, chickpeas

Cereals and grains – basmati, brown, black or wild rice, rice noodles, rice cakes, bulgur and durum wheat, raw oats, quinoa, rye, amaranth, barley, tapioca, buckwheat, kamut, millet, semolina, sorghum, spelt, triticale

Vegetables - sweet potato, onions, fresh ginger and garlic

Cans – baked beans, tuna, salmon, sardines, asparagus, corn

Other – Peanut butter, nut spreads, high quality protein powder

Condiments – spices, dried herbs, black pepper, mustard, tamari sauce, vinegar, onion flakes, seaweed or Celtic salt,* rapadura or brown sugar
Coconut and extra virgin olive oil and sprays

Fridge

Plenty of fresh vegetables, meats, raw nuts and seeds, natural yoghurt, eggs, butter
White cheese - bocconcini, cottage cheese, buffalo mozzarella

Fresh milk, unsweetened almond milk

Fresh herbs, Asian pastes, homemade dressings

Freezer

Frozen peas, vegetables and blueberries

Wheat free breads, homemade soups and extra meals

Fruit Bowl

Lemons, limes, apples, oranges, tomatoes, avocadoes, berries, mangoes and pineapple

*Seaweed and Celtic salts contain many vital minerals and have not been processed, so they still contain essential nutrients such as iodine and iron. Just watch your daily intake of sodium.

Once you are more prepared with your shopping, you can improve the quality of foods you eat by eating more fresh food rather than canned. Take one step at a time to improve your diet so that it sticks forever. If you are actually TAKING ACTION in a simple way, you will establish the habits. Then, you can step things up a little.

With these basic ingredients in your kitchen, you can now create your meal plans and purchase what you need for the meals you have chosen.

TIP: Fresh herbs add fantastic flavour to most meals. Grow your own for great variety all year round! Coriander, parsley, basil, thyme, rosemary and sage – the list goes on!

Stock the kitchen

Stack cans and packets so that you can see them all and arrange foods in similar categories. It may sound pedantic, but it all helps to make better choices if all your healthy options are accessible, rather than at the back of the pantry. Have a wide range to ensure you can eat whatever you feel like at the time that's healthy.

Top Tips

- Keep the pantry and fridge well stocked

- Plan meals ahead of time

- Shop once a week at your supermarket, butcher and health food store

- Cook extra and freeze in portions or use the next day

- Get everyone in the house involved in meal preparation – this will lighten your load and encourages the kids or others to happily eat the prepared meals.

Action

Mind...

Instead of eating while multitasking, try the following strategies:

- Stop all other activities and take a few deep breaths before you start eating.

- Eat without distraction. The television, newspaper or telephone will distract you from getting the signal that you are full. Even music can be distracting. Georgia State University research showed that people eat more when they listen to music.

- Take a moment to enjoy the visual appeal of what you're about to eat, such as the bright, colourful vegetables in a salad or the crispy skin on the salmon.

- Take note of the aroma of your food, savour the first bite and take time to appreciate the flavour of your food before you even start chewing it.

- Pay attention to every mouthful you take: the feeling of creaminess of yogurt, the satisfying crunch of a slice of red capsicum, and the tenderness of a perfectly cooked piece of steak. Savour every mouthful and enjoy eating!

- Put down your fork between bites – this will encourage you to chew well.

- Notice how you feel when you have finished eating. If you overeat, be aware of the physical and emotional discomfort and create a plan to ensure you don't overeat again.

- Before finishing your plate, allow yourself time to notice if you are beginning to feel satisfied. It actually takes about 20 minutes to feel full.

- Every time you eat, enjoy every mouthful and eat slowly. Think ahead to how great your body feels when you are prepared and eat good foods regularly.

Body...

Enjoy the feeling of eating at the right times. Are you less bloated, more energised and enjoy better moods?

Food...

1. Clean out the pantry
2. Research local vendors
3. Write down the menu for the week
4. Create a shopping list
5. Go shopping
6. Re-stock the pantry, fridge and freezer

What to Eat

"We are indeed much more than what we eat, but what we eat can nevertheless help us to be much more than what we are"
Adelle Davis

With all the information available today, it can be very confusing to know what to eat. Most of us have read countless magazines and books on food and diets, visited internet sites, and spoken to friends and experts about *what* to eat. Everywhere in the media, we see different messages about what we should eat. We hear about super foods, diet foods, foods of the celebrities and what to eat for thin thighs, because diets sell. Our basic common sense way on eating has become confused as the result of misinformation and even over-information. Common sense is a powerful tool: if it doesn't seem right, it probably isn't!

To get in great shape, it is crucial that you become truly aware of what you eat. It's also easier and a much more effective method of weight management than hours of daily exercise! If you ensure that your food intake is healthy and balanced, most of the time you are on your way to the body you want.

So, what do you need to eat for fat loss and vitality?

Get back to basic, real food. You will discover that you already know some of the answers. Eat a wide variety of food in its natural state, or as close to it as possible and you are well on the way to feeling brilliant.

There are three types of macronutrients – carbohydrates, fats and proteins – but the types you eat and how much determines your body fat levels. You need a combination of good quality proteins, carbohydrates and fats with each meal to feel satisfied and energised. Eating poor quality foods is a good recipe for fat gain.

Forget counting calories right now – start thinking about *how you feel* when you eat and the quality of food that you put into your body.

If you can choose organic food as much as possible, you avoid chemicals and lessen the load on your liver. The range of organic produce now available is extensive and more reasonably priced, so buy as much organic fruits, vegetables and meat as possible. Organic foods offer more nutrients and no additives, which is good for your health and your body.

Don't be deceived by healthy looking packaging on products. Manufacturers are presenting their goods in packaging so they *appear* to be healthy! They use browns, greens natural colours and soft fonts, with wording such as 'natural', 'healthy' and 'wholesome' to give you the impression that their product is good for you. It may be healthy, but to discover the truth, read the ingredients list.

Have protein, carbohydrates and fats at each meal

This is the secret to enable you to stay satisfied and still lose the fat.

The type and the amount of proteins, fats and carbohydrates you require is unique to you, so listen to your body. If you feel hungry within an hour of eating or notice a drop in energy, you have miscalculated one of your portions of protein, carbohydrates or fat. To lose the extra fat, stack your plate like the one below.

If you feel that your body needs a bit more or less of a particular nutrient, experiment a little to find the perfect ratio for you.

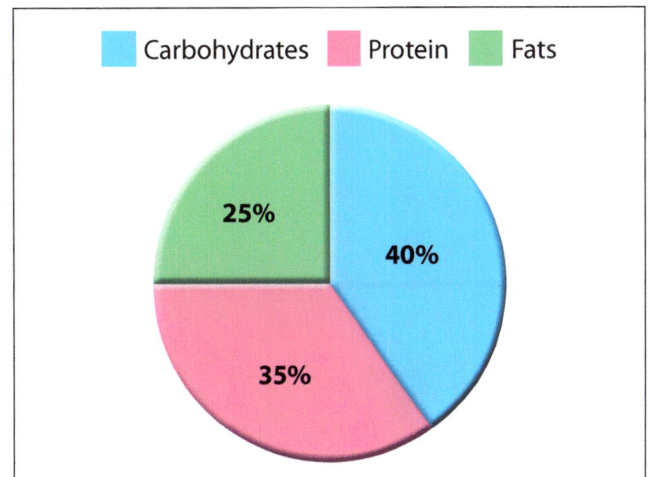

Carbohydrates — Protein — Fats

40% Carbohydrates
35% Protein
25% Fats

What are you eating now?

By filling out a food diary for a week, you will learn a lot about your eating habits. You will become aware of what you actually did eat, as well as how satisfying you found your selection of food. Note down how you feel before and after you eat, and include a rating of your hunger level before and after eating. Rate your hunger level from 1 to 10, 1/10 feeling very full and 10/10 feeling extremely hungry.

With this information, you can refine the quantity and type of food you eat to satisfy all your needs. For example, if you are hungry within an hour of eating breakfast, consider adjusting your portions of carbohydrates, fats and proteins. It's usually a lack of fat or protein if you are soon hungry.

Once your hunger is satisfied between meals and snacks, you will feel great and start losing weight.

Monday

Breakfast – 7am	3 egg omelette with 50g chicken and vegetables
Hunger Pre: 8/10 Post: 1/10	Very satisfied after meal
Snack – 10am	Banana and 100g natural yoghurt
Hunger Pre: 6/10 Post: 2/10	Wasn't starving at snack time for a change!
Lunch – 2:30pm	Ham and salad sandwich on white bread
Hunger Pre: 8/10 Post: 6/10	Very hungry as I ate lunch an hour after I started feeling hungry Not satisfied with white bread and small amount of protein. Was starving again an hour afterwards!

FOOD DIARY	Mon	Tues	Wed	Thur	Fri	Sat	Sun
Breakfast							
Hunger							
Pre:							
Post:							
Snack							
Hunger							
Pre:							
Post:							
Lunch							
Hunger							
Pre:							
Post:							
Snack							
Hunger							
Pre:							
Post:							
Dinner							
Hunger							
Pre:							
Post:							

Notes:

How Much Food?

Once you have mastered the ingredients of a healthy diet, it may be necessary to monitor your portion size to continue losing the fat. Even if the food you are eating is of the highest quality, it is still possible to eat too much.

Some small, conscious reductions in the amount you eat could be the solution for you. This doesn't mean dieting or severely restricting your caloric intake. That can lead to weight gain. It simply means turning your attention to the amount of good quality food your body needs each day. With a little experimentation, this will become automatic as you learn how much food is required to keep you strong and healthy, while still losing the excess weight. The focus is on listening to your body and fuelling it accordingly, as well as enjoying eating whole foods.

Consider following one of the eating plans we have provided for a while, to keep things simple and ensure your portions are the right size. Also consider the pros and cons of counting calories for fat loss and decide whether this technique will work for you.

Counting calories – the pros and cons for fat loss

Counting calories or kilojoules is a widespread obsession for many women in today's society. Every time I visit a fitness club, I hear women discussing how many calories they burnt in their session, rather than what they physically achieved or how good they felt.

Counting calories or kilojoules as a weight management strategy is actually ineffective for many women. Firstly, it's a boring and time-consuming task. The formula for working out the energy required to burn particular foods, along with the differences in people's basal metabolic rates, makes it difficult to correctly use the strategy.

Secondly, it can promote an unhealthy relationship with food, as anything with a high caloric value is considered bad. Thirdly, taken on face value, it takes a lot of output to use all the calories in a simple snack, which can be demoralising. If you ate a sausage roll

(450 calories or 1881kJs) you would need to walk for 1.5 hours to burn it off! This is not very motivating.

However, there are times when counting calories certainly helps. Once you have mastered your mind and its relationship to food and your body, and have learnt how, when and what to eat, you may want to go that little bit further for maximum fat loss results.

To estimate how many calories you need, you can use this simple formula. To get your calorie range, convert your weight in kilograms to pounds, and then multiply this by 10 and 12.

Based on a 60kg woman who does moderate exercise 3-5 times a week		
Convert kg to pounds	60kg x 2.2	= 132 pounds
Multiply by 10-12 calories	132 x 10	= 1,320 calories
	132 x 12	= 1,584 calories

This person should have a daily intake between about 1,300 and 1,580 calories per day, broken up into 3 meals and 2-3 snacks. Experiment a little to see how your body responds. You may find that you need to adjust your food portions.

TIP: Don't go below 1,200 calories per day as you will sabotage your fat loss and risk not getting adequate nutrients.

Consider whether counting calories will positively motivate you to drop the last bit of weight or alternatively lead you to restrict your food intake, depress you and ultimately sabotage your efforts.

Cravings

Cravings can be a major obstacle to your success if they cause you to overeat or make regular unhealthy foods choices. Wouldn't it be great to be rid of them forever?

Interestingly, sugar cravings are reduced when you cut back your sugar intake, so start by eliminating the sugar you won't miss too much. Depending on how addicted you are to sugar, chose a method you know you can stick to. If you love the thought of sugar, try cutting out the hidden sugars first. For example, there is sugar in cereals, baked beans, savoury sauces, soups and many other foods that you might not think have sugar added. Read the list of ingredients, and ensure that sugar is not on the list, or is at least closer to the end. If you can eliminate all of the refined sugar in your diet, go for it! You will feel better within days and have more energy, less mood swings and the cravings will probably disappear. If not, adopt a few of the strategies below.

How to Beat Cravings

1. **Reduce your refined carbohydrate and sugar intake**

2. **Reduce stress and other emotional triggers**

3. **Exercise**

4. **Take a chromium and/or glutamine supplement**

5. **Eat regularly, with adequate protein and fat**

Carbohydrates

Carbohydrates in their natural state are highly nutritious and vital to good health. They are the major fuel source of the body and provide vitamins, minerals and fibre. They can also play a major role in fat loss.

However, the modern diet is inundated with processed and refined carbohydrates which contain little, if any, nutritional value. The excessive consumption of these foods leads to a poor state of health, promotes obesity, diabetes and many other diseases.

Our supermarkets are filled with processed breads, cereals and snack foods. It can be overwhelming just visiting the processed food aisles. With the variety of carbohydrate options available so enormous, many of us are consuming more carbohydrates than ever. The low fat craze which still continues, encourages even more consumption of processed carbohydrates.

Recently, health experts have been advising us to reduce our excessive consumption of processed carbohydrates - which is sound advice. However, some people are taking it to the extreme by dropping all carbohydrates from the diet. It's all quite confusing hey!?

Let's get it straight then, it's not the carbohydrates themselves that are the problem, it's the QUALITY of our carbohydrate intake. Complex, starchy carbohydrates are actually pretty hard to overdose on. The fibre and nutrient content provides satiety and the flavours are satisfying enough - so we just need *more* of this type.

The Goodness of Complex Carbohydrates

The carbohydrates to consume for health and fat loss are complex carbohydrates, found in whole grains, vegetables, beans, pulses and the natural sugars found in fruit and milk. Complex or starchy carbohydrates take longer to break down and digest and provide energy and satiety for a longer duration. They assist with digestion and haven't been refined, stripped of nutrients or altered in any way. Nature provides a healthy bundle of nutrients to provide all of your carbohydrate requirements. Why complicate things?

Simple Carbohydrates - Simply Sugar

Simple carbohydrates are refined carbohydrates and simple sugars which are transported quickly into the blood stream as glucose and provide an instant source of energy. They are found in white flour products like bread and pasta, most breakfast cereals and all things sweet – confectionery, muesli bars, cakes and biscuits, soft drinks, juices, jam and honey.

Simple carbohydrates are needed in small quantities for normal functioning and in greater amounts during intensive endurance training. Most of us get an adequate dose of carbohydrates from natural sources, such as fruit, milk and honey. The problem lies in the overuse (or misuse) of refined sugars, which leads to poor health and weight gain.

Simple carbohydrates and sugars are broken down by the body and used in exactly the same way as if you ate a teaspoon of sugar out of the sugar bowl. So unless you are an endurance athlete, eliminate the simple carbohydrates and increase the amount of good quality carbohydrates in your diet. You will feel great and lose the excessive fat too.

Sweet Seduction

On average, Australians consume 53kg of sugar each year, or around 29 teaspoons of sugar (both added and natural) each day. Of the total sugar we eat, 75% comes from packaged and pre-prepared foods and drinks. And we love our soft drinks! The consumption of soft drinks in Australia has increased 30% in a decade.

Although many of us aim to minimise added sugars in our diet, it isn't always easy, as it has so many names! It is listed on food labels in many different forms - I have discovered over 60 different words that all mean the same thing – sugar!

Some foods contain more sugar than you may think…	
600 ml bottle soft drink	15 tsp of sugar
250 ml apple juice	5 tsp of sugar
1 tbsp tomato sauce	1.5 tsp of sugar
1 serving of Special K	1.5 tsp of sugar

The fake stuff can make you fat and sick

Artificial sweeteners include products such as NutraSweet, Sugarine, Equal and Splenda and may also include high fructose corn syrup. They are more addictive and toxic than real sugar, and actually increase sugar cravings as your body hasn't consumed any REAL sugar so still desires the 'sugar fix'.

These products diminish your sensitivity to naturally sweet tasting foods as the fake stuff is so concentrated – between 180 and 600 times sweeter than sugar. Some artificial sweeteners also contain aspartame, which can cause headaches, abdominal pains, fatigue and depression.

Use natural unrefined sweeteners such as honey, natural maple syrup or rapadura sugar. Rapadura sugar is the dried natural juice of the sugar cane and it retains all the vitamins and minerals naturally available. It's available in health food stores.

Is the Glycaemic Index important?

The Glycaemic Index (GI) is a measure of the effects of carbohydrates on blood sugar levels. A high GI indicates a food that is rapidly absorbed by the body. High GI foods can affect blood sugar levels and weight, and include potatoes, white rice, rice cakes and crackers, white bread and corn flakes.

A low GI indicates a food that is slowly absorbed, so your body is more likely to use it for fuel, rather than store it as fat. Low GI foods include oats, wholegrain breads, most vegetables, fruit, beans, dairy and nuts. Low GI foods tend to keep you fuller for longer. Notice how you feel satisfied for longer if you eat a slice of wholegrain bread rather than white bread? The good news is that most of the starchy types of vegetables which help keep you full have a low GI rating.

The GI rating of foods can be confusing, as for example bran flakes have a high GI, but All Bran has a low GI. And some unhealthy foods have a low GI. So don't put too much importance on GI ratings, instead be aware of what you are eating so you stay fuelled for longer. If you are diabetic or an endurance athlete who needs to refuel quickly after intense training, the GI rating can be a useful tool.

Excessive consumption of simple carbohydrates will make you fat.

Consume around 40% of your daily intake from good quality carbohydrates

Facts on Fats

For thousands of years, obesity was rarely seen. It was not until the 20th century that it became so common that in 1997, the World Health Organisation (WHO) formally recognised obesity as a global epidemic. In 2007, the WHO found that 67.4% of Australian adults were overweight and just over 20% were obese. If current trends continue, these figures will keep rising.

In the 1950's a questionable study by Dr Ancel Keys in the United States changed the developed world's view on saturated fats, blaming them for our rising state of poor health. The study concluded that saturated fats were responsible for the soaring rates of heart disease in the USA. While many questioned his findings, Dr Keys' conclusions were accepted as fact by the American Heart Association, and by the medical community at large. We were told to cut our saturated fat intake and increase the consumption of man-made vegetable oils and margarine, as well as eating less total fat.

Numerous studies since then have given us plenty of reason to question the accuracy of this data, and the statistics show that despite our efforts, we are fatter than ever. In the 1960's, fats and oils made up around 45% of the calories in the American diet, and only 13% of people were obese. Now, only 33% of calories are from fats and oils, and 34% of Americans are obese.

Similarly, heart disease was blamed on the consumption of saturated fats, but it is more common that ever, despite the widespread change to polyunsaturated fats in our diet.

Fat is actually highly nutritious and aids fat loss, but it is important to be aware of which fats are good for you and which fats to avoid.

The Good Stuff
There are two types of healthy fats found naturally in food: saturated and unsaturated.

Saturated Fats
Saturated fats are found mostly in animals and tropical plant oils and are a rich source of vitamins. They are essential to the human body, and in fact, the human brain and breast milk are made up of 50% saturated fat. Saturated fats are highly stable, which means that they do not normally go rancid, even when heated for cooking purposes.

Unsaturated fats
Unsaturated fats are found in both animal and plants and are liquid at room temperature. Your body cannot make these essential fatty acids, so you must obtain them through your diet. The two types of EFA's are omega-3 and omega-6 fatty acids.

Omega-3 fatty acids are an essential polyunsaturated fat, whereas its cousin Omega-6 is not so needed. Our diet often contains far greater amounts of Omega-6 than Omega-3. This is due to our high grain and vegetable oil intake, as well as the diet of the animals we consume. Modern farming techniques have reduced the amount of Omega-3 naturally found in food. Eggs, for instance, are naturally rich in Omega-3, provided the eggs come from free ranging chickens that eat a natural diet of insects and worms.

Studies at the University of South Australia found that taking Omega-3 fish oil in combination with moderate aerobic exercise boosts weight loss. The Omega-3 fish oils activate the fat-burning enzymes and increase the metabolic rate. Omega-3 fats also play a role in assisting conditions such as heart disease, Alzheimer's, cancers, inflammatory diseases, depression and diabetes.

Fats to Avoid

Throughout history, cultures all over the world have used saturated fats, not polyunsaturated fats, as their main fat for cooking. Heart disease rates began to increase AFTER people started replacing natural fats with polyunsaturated fats such as vegetable oils.

Polyunsaturated Omega-6 Fatty Acids

Polyunsaturated Omega-6 fatty acids are essential fatty acids, however most of us consume far in excess of what is needed.

Vegetable oils made from corn and grains require extensive processing in order to lengthen their shelf life and improve texture and flavour. They undergo processes such as hexane solvent baths, bleaching, neutralisation and deodorisation. In comparison, the more healthy choice of olive oil is extracted by simply pressing olives!

When polyunsaturated Omega-6 fatty acids are exposed to heat, air and light they easily turn rancid. They then oxidise and spit free radicals throughout the body. These rancid oils are a major source of free radicals in our diet. They can promote or cause the development of diseases, such as cancer, rheumatism, Alzheimer's, arthritis and cataracts. They cause oxidative damage and promote the ageing process.

Cooking with Oils

Oils high in **polyunsaturated** fats turn rancid easily when heated (corn, soybean, safflower and sunflower oils).

Oils high in **monounsaturated** fats can tolerate quite high heat during cooking (olive, sesame, peanut, rice bran and some types of sunflower oil).

Oils high in **saturated** fats are very stable and most suitable for high heat cooking, such as deep frying (coconut and palm oil, and various types of animal fat).

To ensure you are using good quality, non-rancid vegetable oils, buy cold-pressed oils that have been extracted without the use of high heat or chemicals. They should be stored in dark bottles, kept away from heat and preferably be unrefined and organic.

Trans Fats

Trans fats are man-made and were created to keep unstable vegetable oils stable. This was a commercially viable discovery for food manufacturers, as these partially hydrogenated oils (PHOs) don't spoil easily and they can withstand repeated heating without breaking down. This allows for easier transportation, longer shelf life and lower cost than animal fats. Over the last several decades, PHOs have become a mainstay in margarines, baked goods, pre-prepared meals, snack foods and much more.

Trans fats consumption has now been strongly linked to increasing the risk of cardiovascular heart disease. It is estimated that between 30,000 and 100,000 cardiac deaths per year in the United States are attributable to the consumption of trans fats. They also promote obesity, insulin resistance, stroke, diabetes and depression.

To avoid trans fats, check the ingredients list for hydrogenated oil, partially hydrogenated oils, hydrogenised vegetable oil, vegetable shortening, shortened fats and oils.

Monoglycerides and diglycerides are classed as emulsifiers, but they may also contain trans-fatty acids. This means a food may be labelled as having 0% trans fat, yet still contain trans fat from Monoglycerides and diglycerides. Sneaky hey!

Three Fat Myths

Butter is bad for you, margarine is good for you
Butter comes from simply natural ingredients mixed together – the body likes it that way and can easily digest it.

When manufacturers created a butter alternative, they added a whole lot of extra ingredients besides just trans fats! Ingredients list for butter - milk fat, cream and salt

Ingredients list for margarine - edible oils, salt or potassium chloride, antioxidant (320), emulsifiers (soy lecithin, 471), preservative 202, food acid, flavours, Vitamins (A, D) colour (beta carotene or 102) 160b – annatto.

Cholesterol is bad for your health

Yes, that's right; cholesterol is back in the good books after an unfair bashing over the years! Cholesterol is a natural substance within the body, is necessary for the production of some hormones, assists with the absorption of fat from food and occurs in very high concentrations in the brain and nervous system. It's time to reconsider what we hear and think about cholesterol.

More than One Egg a Day is Bad for Your Cholesterol Levels

The egg is one of the few foods to naturally contain vitamin D. A yolk contains most of the recommended daily intake of cholesterol; however, one study indicates the human body may not absorb much cholesterol from eggs. All the egg's vitamin A, D, and E are found in the egg yolk. Most of us could do with all the egg's natural nutrients!

	GOOD FATS	BAD FATS
Oils and butter	Coconut, palm, palm kernels, sesame seeds, peanuts	Hydrogenated, partially hydrogenated vegetable oils Industrially processed vegetable oils (corn, soybean, safflower, sunflower) Fats and oils heated to very high temperatures
Nut oils	Unheated organic nut oils: macadamia, walnut olives and its oil (cold pressed) avocado and its oil, krill oil, chia and inca inchi oils	Heated nut oils
Fish and their oils	All fish, especially oily fish (e.g. salmon, trout, tuna, herring), lightly pan-fried or oven baked High quality fish oil tablets from pure sources (seek advice on this)	Deep fried fish Synthetically-produced or farmed fish and their oils (seek advice on this)
Nuts	Raw nuts e.g. almonds, cashews, macadamias, Brazil, hazelnuts or pecans	Roasted nuts
Meats	Grass fed meats	Grain-fed meat, processed meats
Eggs	Organic pastured eggs	Grain-fed eggs
Pastries	Home-made, trans fat free pastries and cakes	Cakes, pastries, biscuits made with trans fats
Dairy	Butter, cream, hard cheese, milk	Margarine

Consume around 25% of your daily intake from healthy fat sources

Protein

Protein provides the building blocks for the body to construct and repair tissues such as muscle, hair, skin, and connective tissue, which make up about 16% of our total body weight. Protein is vital for immunity and also plays a pivotal role in muscle mass development and fat loss.

Protein-rich foods from animal sources are full of nutrients. Lean red meat is the richest source of iron and zinc, and it is better absorbed by our bodies than from plant foods. Animal products are excellent sources of vitamin B12, a nutrient not found in plant foods, and fish and seafood are the richest sources of Omega-3 fats.

How much are we REALLY eating?

Unfortunately, we often unintentionally don't get enough protein in our diet. As a result of the low fat craze (which has lasted over 20 years!) we have increased our carbohydrate intake without enough consideration of our protein consumption. Guidelines, thankfully, are beginning to change as experts realise our protein intake is now inadequate.

Many women I see have a very low protein intake and high body fat levels. This may be partly attributable to the body breaking down its own muscle tissue stores in order to meet its requirements, which results in muscle mass loss and fat gain. Fat tissue also has a much lower resting metabolic rate, so the higher your level of muscle mass the more energy burnt while you are at rest.

Consider when you normally eat most of your protein - is it at dinner time? Try spreading out your protein intake throughout the day, particularly at breakfast. After fasting all night, your body may start drawing on muscle tissue for fuel if you don't replenish its protein stores first thing in the morning. A protein-rich breakfast will also help regulate your appetite all day.

Five Power-Packed Reasons to Eat Protein for Fat Loss

1. Keeps you fuller for longer, promoting weight loss
2. Uses more energy to digest and assimilate
3. Builds muscle, prevents muscle wastage and boosts metabolism
4. Protein aids recovery from exercise and builds muscle tissue
5. Protein reduces the risk of disease

Research shows a diet high in lean protein sources reduces blood pressure, 'bad' cholesterol levels and triglycerides better than a traditional high-carbohydrate low-protein diet. Diets rich in protein can also help prevent obesity, osteoporosis and diabetes.

Protein also helps build muscle, which is the metabolic furnace that burns fat. If you are trying to lose weight, you must maintain healthy muscle. Even at rest, your body needs protein to repair and build new tissues, make haemoglobin and protect you from disease. These processes all require adequate protein intake – so eat up! For weight loss, aim for 4-5 serves (every 3-4 hours) of protein daily.

Consume around 35% of your daily intake from lean protein sources

Good Food Guide

CARBOHYDRATES
~ 40% of Plate, 3-5 serves daily

Fibrous vegetables (1 serve = 1 cup)	Asparagus, green beans, bok choy broccoli, Brussels sprouts, cabbage, capsicum, celery cauliflower, cucumber, leeks, lettuce, mushrooms, onions, spinach, squash, snow peas, tomato, turnip, zucchini
Starchy, high carbohydrate vegetables (1 serve = ½ cup)	Carrots, corn, pumpkin, sweet potato, lentils, peas Beans – cannellini, borlotti, red kidney, chickpeas, lima, butter, black beans, black eyed peas
Grains (1 serve = ½ cup)	Rice – brown, black, wild, basmati Breads – whole grain, multi grain and gluten free Pasta – rice and corn varieties, preferably gluten free Gluten free grains and flours - amaranth, arrowroot, buckwheat, coconut flour, corn flour, lentil flour, malt-free rice and corn breakfast cereals, millet, polenta, potato flour, rice bran, rice flour, sago, sorghum, soy flour, tapioca, oats
Fruit (1 serve = 1 medium piece)	

PROTEINS
~ 35% of Plate, 3-5 serves daily

Meat – grass-fed (1 serve = 100g/3.5oz)	Red meat and poultry
Fresh fish – (1 serve = 115g/4oz)	White fish – flathead, snapper, barramundi, perch etc. Salmon, tuna and trout – wild, not farmed Shellfish – prawns, crab, lobster
Tinned fish (1 serve ~185g tin)	Sardines, tuna, salmon, herring, mackerel, anchovies
Dairy (1 serve)	Eggs, 3-4 whites, 1 yolk Cheese, low fat, 75g Cottage cheese, ½ cup
Soy Products (1 serve)	Tofu, ½ cup Soy beans, cooked, 1 cup
Protein powder (1 serve = 30g)	(useful for fuelling around exercise and as an emergency snack) Other foods that are high in protein include: quinoa, yoghurt (natural), cow's milk (low fat), soy milk, quark cheese (low fat), parmesan cheese, beans and split peas

FATS
~ 25% of Plate, 3 serves daily with meals

Oils, 1 tbsp Nuts, 15 Seeds, 1-2 tbsp e.g. sesame, pumpkin, sunflower	Olives, 10 Avocado, ¼ Coconut, shredded, 2 tbsp
Dairy	Butter, 2 tsp Cream cheese, reduced fat, 2 tbsp Cream, reduced fat, 2 tbsp
Animal Products	Bacon, pancetta, bresaola, 2 slices Oily fish, 100g

Food Labelling

Food labels provide most of the information needed to discover what is in the packaged foods we eat. The labels include the nutrition information as well as the actual ingredients list. The nutrition information label allows you to compare the amount of energy, fat, sugar, fibre, salt (and often vitamins and minerals) in different products per serve or per 100g.

This information can be useful, however many people find it confusing as they don't know what the appropriate or ideal amounts should be. So even after reading the label, you don't have all the information you need to make an informed, healthy choice. To give you a little clarity, the blue box below indicates how much of each nutrient we should be aiming for.

NUTRITION INFORMATION

Servings per pack: 5 Serving size: 22g	Average Quantity per serving	per 100g
Energy	384kJ 92Cal	1744kJ 417Cal
Protein	0.8g	3.5g
Fat, total	1.9g	8.7g
- saturated	0.8g	3.5g
Carbohydrate	17.0g	77.3g
- sugars	7.2g	32.8g
Dietary Fibre	1.3g	6.0g
Sodium	26mg	117mg
Gluten	0mg	0mg

Ideal Amounts

Fat – less than 10g fat per 100g

Sugar – less than 50% of the total carbohydrate

Fibre – more than 10g of dietary fibre per 100g

Salt – less than 150mg of sodium per serve

Read the ingredients list

The list of ingredients is more useful and informative, as it states **what is actually in** the product. The list is written with the largest ingredient first, down to the minor ingredients. If the list is long, with lots of numbers and chemical-sounding names, it's probably not very healthy.

Food manufacturers make plenty of claims to help sell the product, but often don't tell us what the food is actually made from.

A popular cereal brands has the following messages on its packaging:

* 98% fat free
* Heart Foundation tick of approval
* High in fibre
* Contains six essential vitamins and minerals
* Good source of wholegrain

But the following ingredients list suggests it's not so healthy, with many additives and a wide variety of different types of sugars.

Cereals (60%) [Wholegrains (51%) (wheat, oats), corn, wheat bran], fruit pieces [fruit concentrates (apple, apricot (0.5%), mango, banana, pineapple juice), invert sugar, sugar, humectant (glycerol), wheat fibre, vegetable fat, maize starch, acidity regulator (330), gelling agent (pectin), flavour, colours (annatto, beta carotene), emulsifier (sunflower lecithin)], sugar, fruit (7%) [sultanas, freeze dried apricot (0.5%)], corn maltodextrin, minerals (calcium phosphate, ferrous lactate, iron), glucose syrup, salt, barley malt extract, honey, humectant (glycerol), emulsifier (471), wheat dextrose, vitamins (niacin, thiamin, riboflavin, folate).

Why not make your own muesli with oats, quinoa, seeds and nuts? You will know exactly what you are eating and save some money too!

Additives

According to Julie Eady, an expert in food additives, "The so-called 'healthy average Australian diet' can easily provide you with over 100 toxic food chemicals each day. Many of these are suspect carcinogens and proven to cause nervous system damage, hyperactivity, damage to babies, children, pregnant and breastfeeding women."

Many food additives that are banned in other countries because of health concerns are still available in Australian products. Some good news is that most supermarkets in Australia, including Aldi and Woolworths, have now at least removed all artificial colours from their foods.

There are plenty of safe additives, however some are best avoided, listed here with their corresponding numbers.

Additives to avoid
COLOURS
102,104,110,122,123,124,127,129, 132,133,142,143, 151,155, 160b (annatto)

PRESERVATIVES
- Sorbates 200-203
- Benzoates 210-213
- Sulphites 220-228
- Nitrates, nitrites 249-252
- Propionates 280-283

SYNTHETIC ANTIOXIDANTS
- Gallates 310-312
- TBHQ, BHA, BHT 319-321

FLAVOUR ENHANCERS
- Glutamates 620-625
- Ribonucleotides 627, 631, 635
- Hydrolysed Vegetable Protein (HVP)

ARTIFICIAL FLAVOURS
Artificial flavours do not include numbers on food labels because they are closely guarded trade secrets. When the word 'flavours' appears on the ingredients list this means they are man-made, even when the label says 'natural flavours'.

For more information visit: www.fedup.com.au, www.chemicalmaze.com or www.additivealert.com.au. You can also buy a handy application for your phone from www.chemicalmaze.com to refer to in the supermarket.

Eating Out

At a wonderful Italian café near my house, there is a cabinet showcasing a wide range of gorgeous paninis and pastas for lunch. On my initial scan, it seemed like it might be difficult to get a meal at this café that was balanced with proteins, fats and carbohydrates. I asked a few questions and it turned out there were lots of options for balanced meals. They had homemade baked beans, lentil soup, cooked chicken, roast vegetables, salads and plenty more.

Don't be afraid to ask questions when eating out; you may even be able to create your own dish to ensure you get a balanced meal.

Eating socially can be healthy if you think ahead and choose a little wisely. That way, you can enjoy yourself without feeling like you are missing out.

TIPS

- Choose restaurants that produce fresh, healthy meals and are flexible with menu changes.
- Ask for dressings and sauces on the side.
- Don't eat all the bread and extras before your meal – enjoy the meal you ordered.
- Choose dishes that are clean and natural.
- Include a little rice, if desired, in Asian restaurants, but aim to eat more vegetables rather than filling up on rice.

FOODS TO EAT

International	Thai	Japanese	Chinese	Italian	Indian
Grilled fish, steak, steamed vegetables, chicken breast and salad, oysters, mussels, calamari, scallops	Rice paper rolls, soups, steamed fish, vegetables, salads	Sashimi, sushi, salads, yakitori, seaweed, mushrooms, ramen soups	Soups, steamed vegetables dishes, stir-fries	Minestrone soup, fish chicken, buffalo mozzarella Thin-based pizzas with lean meat and lots of vegetables	Sautéed spinach, paneer, chicken tikka or tandoori, baked or grilled fish, dahl and vegetable dishes

FOODS TO AVOID

International	Thai	Japanese	Chinese	Italian	Indian
Dressings, heavy sauces fried foods	Fried foods, creamy dishes	Deep fried dishes such as tempura, dumplings	Most starters, deep fried foods and sticky sauces	Thick based pizzas, toppings like bacon, salami, extra cheese, creamy pastas	Creamy sauces, deep fried and oily dishes, poppadoms

Sample 5 Day Eating Plan

Day 1	Day 2	Day 3	Day 4	Day 5
Warm water and lemon	Warm water and lemon	Warm water and lemon	Warm water and lemon	Warm water and lemon
BREAKFAST	**BREAKFAST**	**BREAKFAST**	**BREAKFAST**	**BREAKFAST**
Warm egg salad – with spinach leaves, green beans, lentils, capsicum	Oats with berries, natural yoghurt, crushed nuts and seeds	Salmon omelette	Toast with turkey or cottage cheese and avocado	Omelette: turkey, tomato capsicum, asparagus (Mostly egg whites)
SNACK	**SNACK** 1 mandarin and 1 peach	**SNACK**	**SNACK**	**SNACK**
Handful raw nuts and banana	**LUNCH**	Soup – ham and pea	Tin of tuna, spinach	Dip and veg sticks
LUNCH	Soup	**LUNCH**	**LUNCH**	**LUNCH**
Turkey salad	**SNACK**	Soup	Chicken and cannellini bean salad	Beef, salad/veg and brown rice
SNACK	Corn thins - turkey and hummus or avocado	**SNACK**	**SNACK**	**SNACK**
Protein shake	**DINNER**	Corn thins, cottage cheese and mash	Egg and avocado	Soup or protein shake
DINNER	Salmon and mashed roast beetroot or sweet potato	**DINNER**	**DINNER**	**DINNER**
Soup – lentil or chicken and vegetables	**SNACK** – if hungry	Roast Chicken	Steak and vegetables	Flat head tails and veg
SNACK – if hungry	Protein powder, with tsp choc/ cocoa powder (freeze for 15min to make a mousse)	**SNACK** – if hungry	**SNACK** Fruit	**SNACK**
Rooibos tea, piece of fruit		Handful nuts, seeds on natural yoghurt		Yoghurt, walnuts
		2 fish oil tablets daily		

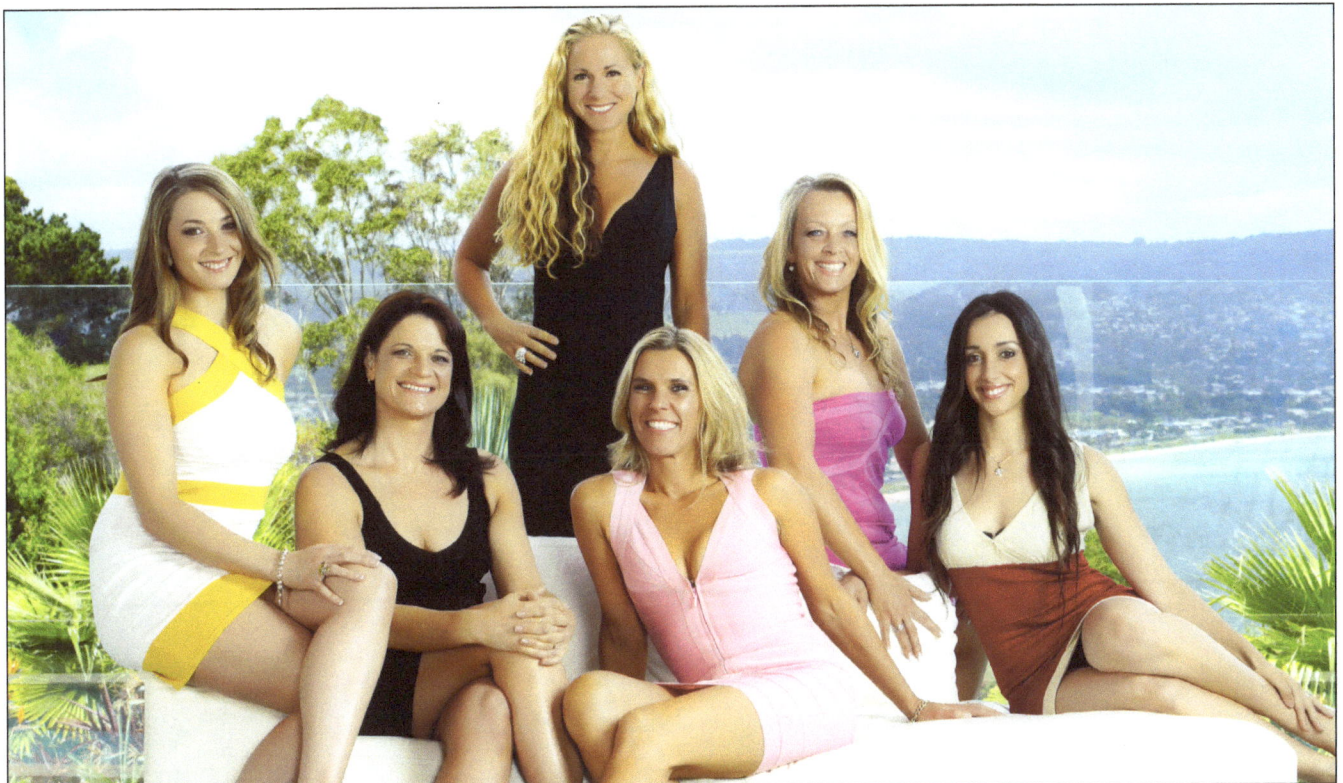

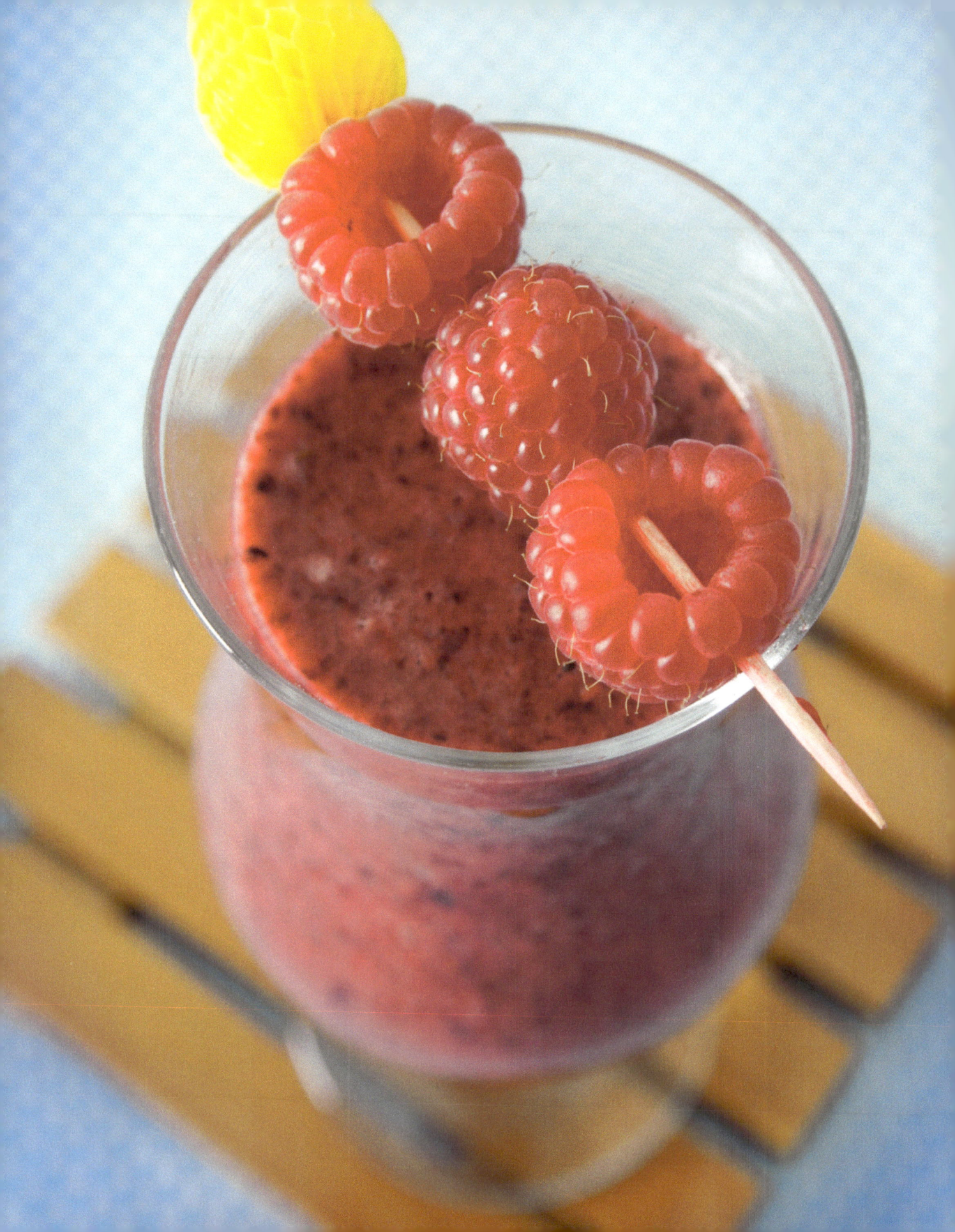

Recipes and Meal Ideas

WARNING!

This is not intended to be a complex recipe chapter, filled with beautiful photos of meals that are difficult to create and never quite turn out like the glossy photos. These are real meals I prepared in my own kitchen, and I'm no chef! They are healthy and tasty meals real women can prepare in a realistic amount of time.

Of course, presenting your dishes beautifully does help you enjoy your meal and even digest it better, as your salivary glands prepare to break down your food at the sight of a nicely presented dish. But sometimes in real life, we only have time to toss all the ingredients together. The main thing is that you have something healthy and tasty on your plate.

Cooking healthy and delicious meals CAN be quick and easy – it's about fresh ingredients, good flavours and the right equipment. Fresh meats, seafood, vegetables and herbs are top priorities. An oven-proof pan is really useful for meats and vegetables.

Check out the simple recipes for some of my favourites - they taste great and are EASY to prepare!

Also keep in mind, it's quite easy to throw some ingredients together to make a healthy meal, quickly. Sometimes a recipe isn't what you need, it's just good ingredients combined!

TIP

Meals and snacks should be eaten when you are hungry. If you are hungry at 11.30am, have your lunch and follow up with a decent snack at around 3pm. If you are not very hungry by dinner time, have a smaller portion.

Breakfast

If you have your pantry and fridge stocked well you can prepare the following breakfasts in a flash.

Very Berry Smoothie
Serves 1

1 scoop vanilla protein powder
¼ cup natural Greek or biodynamic yoghurt
¾ cup fresh or frozen berries, eg blueberries, raspberries and strawberries
2 tbsp LSA (linseed, sunflower seed and almond mix)
½ cup of ice
1 cup water or milk - almond, rice, soy or cows
Blend until smooth and pour into a glass
Top with berries on a skewer

Yoghurt with nuts and berries
Serves 1

1 cup of natural or biodynamic yoghurt
2 tbsp protein powder
½ cup blueberries
Handful almonds
2 tbsp chia seeds
2 tbsp shredded coconut
Cinnamon to taste
Place yoghurt in a bowl and top with all of the ingredients

Homemade Muesli with Yoghurt
Serves 4

2 cups organic rolled oats
¼ cup rice bran
½ cup quinoa flakes
2 tbsp mixed sunflower and sesame seeds
2 tbsp pumpkin seeds
2 tbsp slivered or smashed almonds
1 tbsp chia seeds
100g pitted dates, cranberries or goji berries
Cinnamon and shredded coconut to taste
Mix well and store in an airtight container
Serve with 1 cup natural biodynamic yoghurt or Greek yoghurt

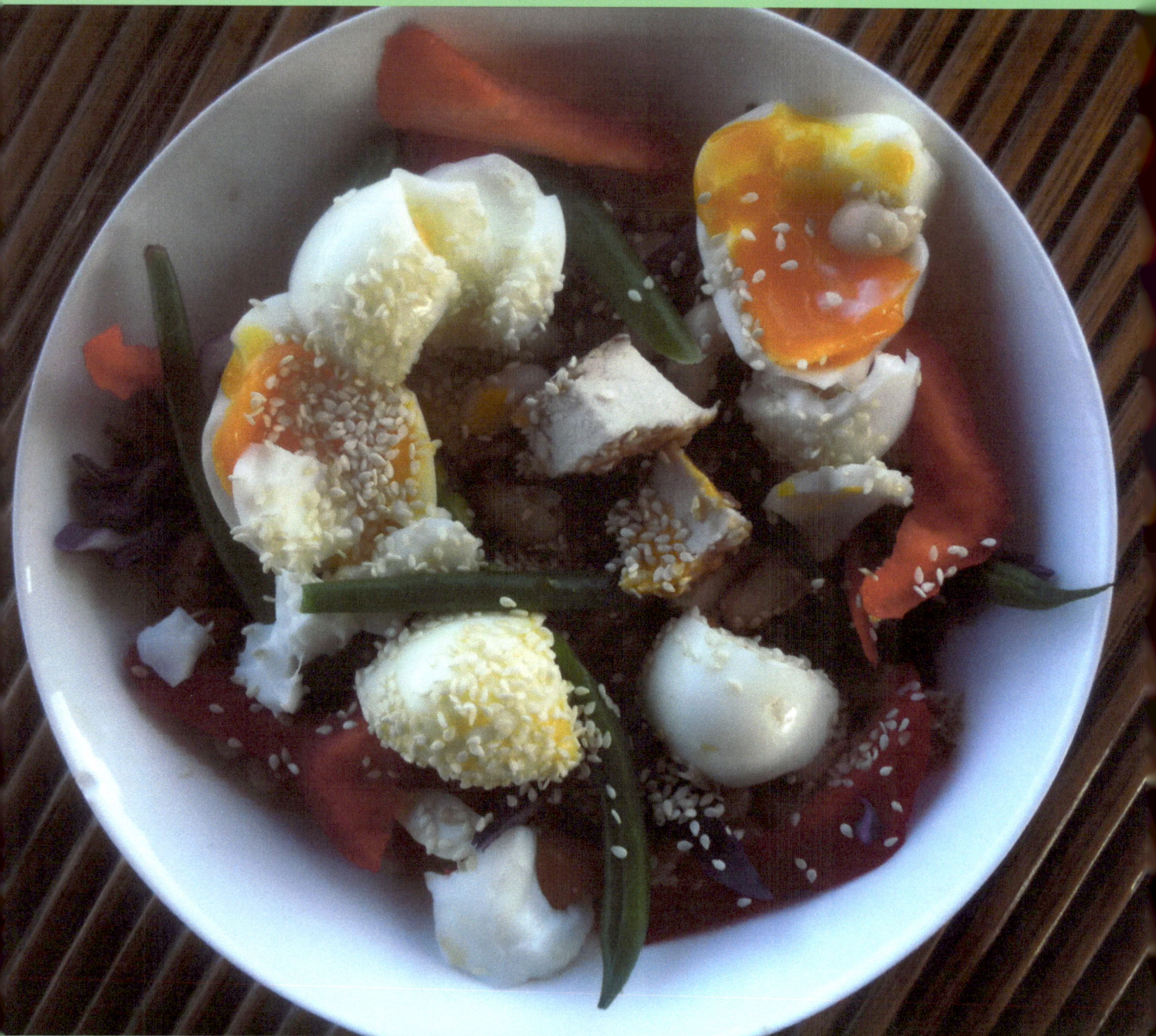

Warm Egg Salad

Serves 1

3 boiled eggs (1-2 yolks)

Large handful of warmed torn spinach leaves

6 sliced green beans

¼ capsicum, sliced

¼ avocado or 3 baby bocconcini, sliced

Combine in a bowl and sprinkle with sesame seeds

MIX IT UP:

Vary this warm breakfast idea by adding or substituting one or two of the following ingredients: left over roast sweet potato or roast beetroot, chicken, cannellini beans or cabbage.

Soft-boiled eggs with steamed asparagus

Serves 1

2 free-range or organic eggs

200g asparagus, trimmed

Salt and freshly ground pepper to taste

Add the eggs to a small pan of water and bring to the boil, add asparagus and boil for 3 minutes.

Place asparagus on a plate and gently squash eggs over the top. Add salt and pepper, if desired.

Omelette

Serves 1

1 onion or spring onion, chopped

100g mushrooms, sliced

4 cherry tomatoes, quartered

100g asparagus, cut into 2cm pieces

¼ capsicum, chopped

1 slice of lean ham, chopped or ¼ cup cottage cheese or light shredded cheese

50g torn baby spinach

4 egg whites

Parsley to garnish

2 tsp oil for cooking

Heat one teaspoon of the oil in an oven-proof frypan, and sauté the onion. Add the mushrooms, tomato, asparagus, capsicum and ham (if using) and cook until soft (3-4 minutes). Season with pepper and sea salt if desired. Add the spinach and cook for one minute.

Whisk the eggs in a bowl. Add the cooked vegetables to the eggs and mix till combined.

Add the rest of the oil to the pan and when hot, pour in the mixture. Add the cheese (if using) and bake in the oven at 200 degrees for 4-5 minutes.

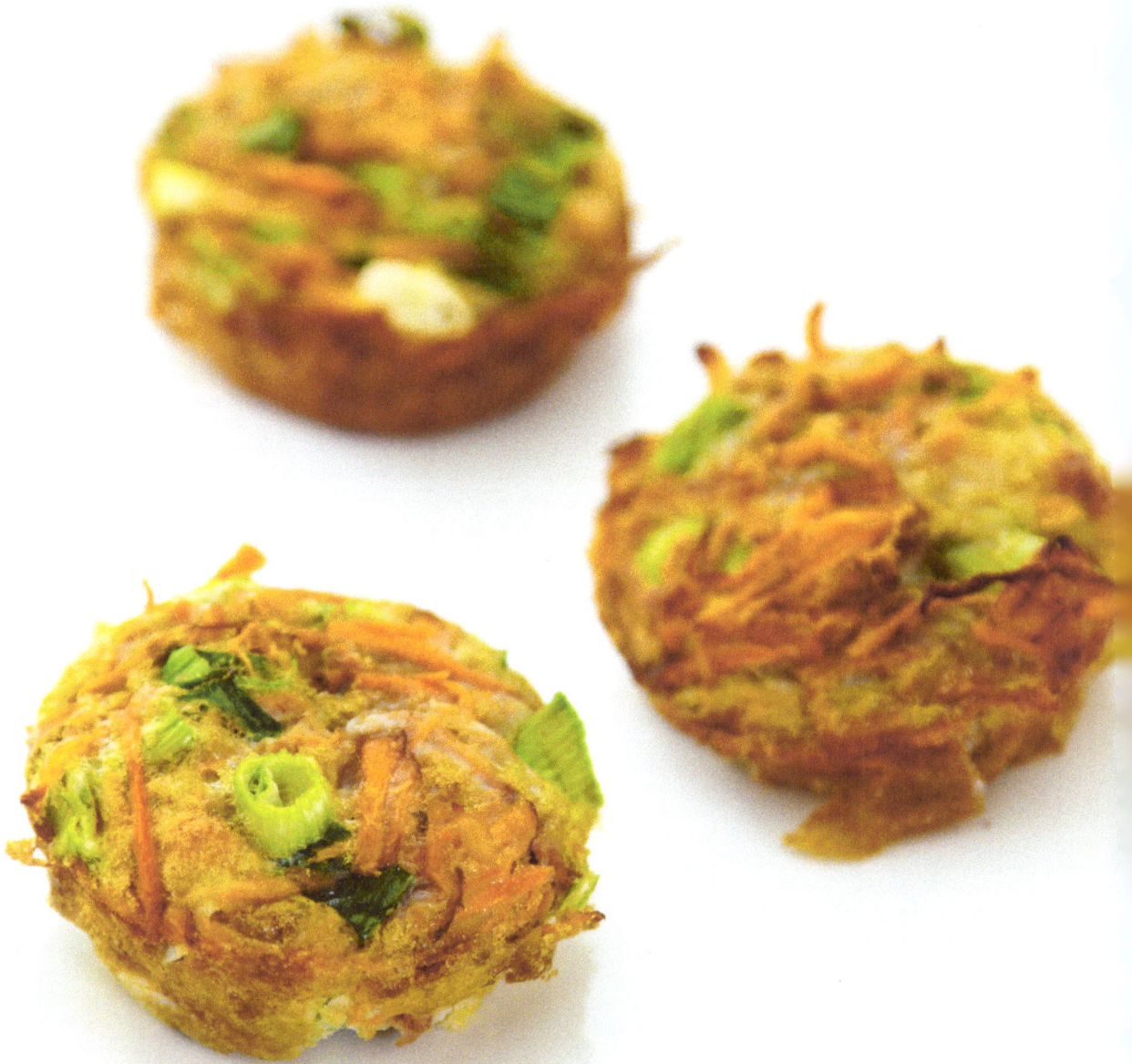

Protein Packed Muffins

Makes 12 muffins (Prepare these the day before for a great breakfast or snack on the run.)

12 large egg whites
2 egg yolks
120g chicken, turkey or smoked salmon, finely chopped
2 cups mixed vegetables - grated zucchini or carrot, finely chopped red onion, red capsicum, asparagus, broccoli and cooked sweet potato
2 handfuls of spinach (or 250g frozen, thawed)
Coriander and parsley, chopped

Whisk eggs in a large bowl then add meat and vegetables. Pour evenly into a greased 12 cup muffin tray.
Cook at 180 degrees for 15-20 minutes.

Apple Cinnamon Pancake

Serves 1

½ cup rolled oats
4 egg whites
½ apple, diced
1 tsp cinnamon

MIX IT UP:
For a HIGH protein breakfast, add 1 scoop of vanilla protein powder.

Combine all ingredients in a bowl until the mixture is smooth. Spray a frying pan with a little olive or coconut oil spray on medium heat. Pour mixture into the pan and cook for 2-3 minutes or until the underside is lightly browned. Turn the pancake over and cook until lightly browned.

Wheat-free or Whole Grain Toast Topped with a selection of:

- smoked salmon, ham or turkey, avocado and tomato
- cottage cheese and tomato
- sardines
- nut spread or peanut butter
- baked beans (preferably home-made)
- leftovers like Italian meat sauce or stew

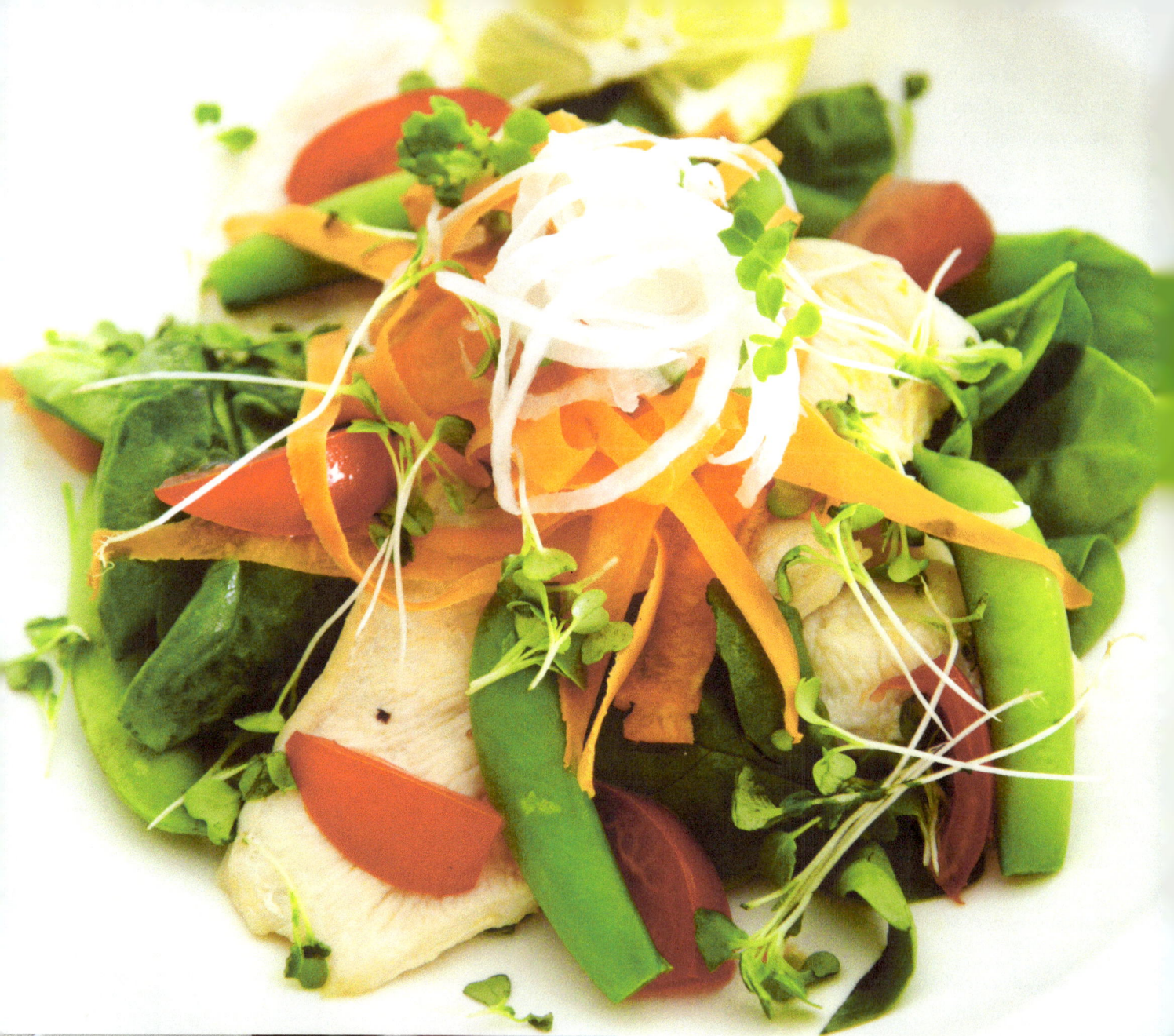

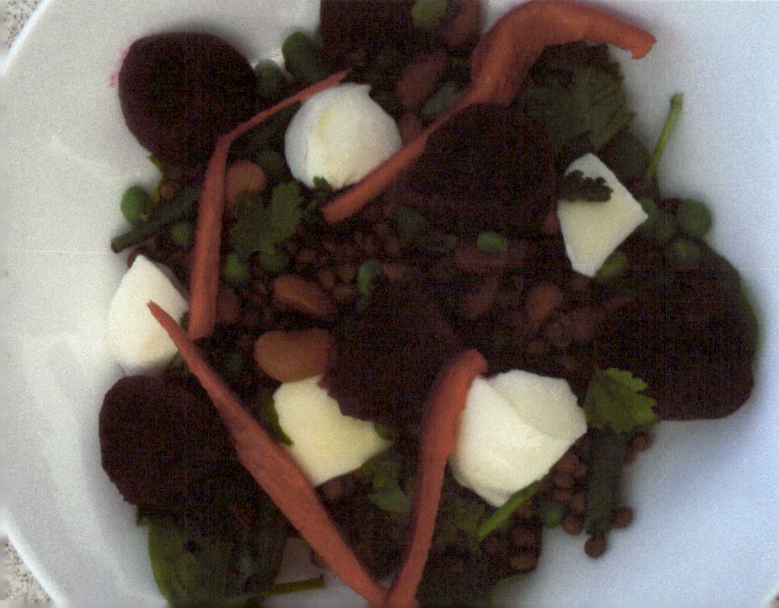

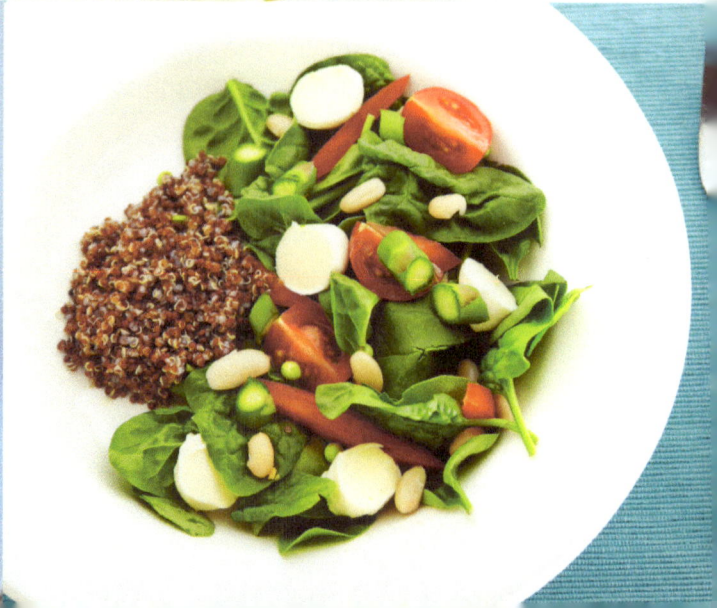

Lunch

Chicken and Sugar Snap Pea Salad
Serves 2

Easy to prepare if you have cooked extra chicken fillets.

2 cooked chicken breast fillets
12 sugar snap peas
8 cherry tomatoes, halved
Handful of baby spinach
¼ avocado, sliced
¼ carrot, grated in long strips

Combine the ingredients in a serving bowl and garnish with micro herbs, shaved radish and a lemon wedge.

Lentils, Borlotti Beans, Baby Beets and Bocconcini Salad
Serves 1

Easy to prepare if you have cooked extra roast baby beets.

Handful of baby spinach leaves
¼ tin brown lentils
Handful of borlotti beans
Handful of fresh peas
3 roast baby beets, halved
4 baby bocconcinis
5 green beans
¼ red capsicums, sliced julienne (thin strips)
Fresh coriander

Place all ingredients except capsicum and coriander in a bowl and warm for around 30 seconds in the microwave on high. (Alternatively, warm the ingredients in a pan on low heat for about 5 minutes, adding spinach last)
Add the capsicum and top with coriander.

MIX IT UP:
You might like to add seeds or a little avocado.

Quinoa, Cannellini Bean and Bocconcini Salad
Serves 2

1 cup of red or white quinoa
2 cups of water
1 stock cube
8 asparagus spears, sliced
Large handful of baby spinach
½ cup cannellini beans
¼ capsicum, sliced
8 cherry tomatoes, quartered
8 baby bocconcini, halved
Drizzle of olive oil

Rinse quinoa in a strainer and transfer to a saucepan. Add water and crushed stock cube then bring to the boil. Reduce to simmer. Cover and cook until water is absorbed (about 15 minutes) or until the quinoa appears translucent. Allow to sit for 5 minutes for a fluffy texture. Steam asparagus and combine with baby spinach, beans, capsicum, tomatoes and bocconcini. Drizzle with olive oil.

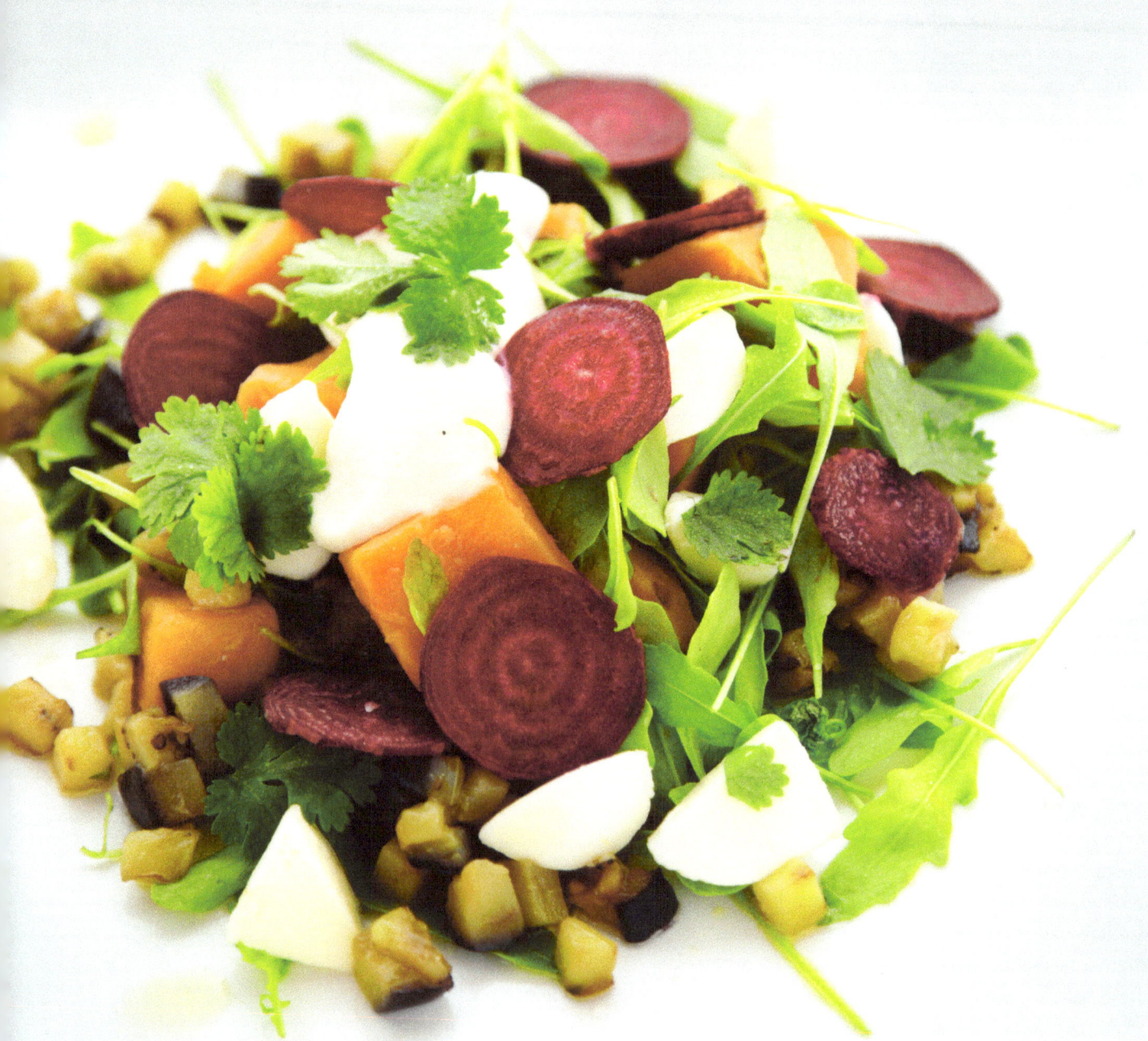

Beetroot, bocconcini and eggplant salad
Serves 2

2 baby beetroots, VERY thinly sliced (a mandolin is the best option)
1 sweet potato, cubed
1 eggplant, diced in small pieces
10 baby bocconcinis
Large handful of baby rocket
Drizzle of olive oil
Coriander as desired

Pre-heat oven to 180 degrees Celsius. Boil sweet potato for 10-15 minutes, or until a knife can cut though it easily. Drain and set aside. Place eggplant on oven-proof tray, spray with oil and bake in the oven for around 15 minutes. While this is baking, slice baby beets thinly and half baby bocconcinis.

Make a bed of eggplant on a plate. Add rocket, sweet potato, beetroot and bocconcini. Drizzle with olive oil and top with coriander.

Tuna and Avocado Salad
Serves 1

95g tin of tuna
Handful of baby spinach, warmed
¼ tin of chickpeas
4 baby Roma tomatoes
¼ avocado, sliced
Handful of cabbage, thinly sliced
Sprinkle of sesame seeds

Blanche or microwave the spinach until wilted.
Combine all ingredients and serve.

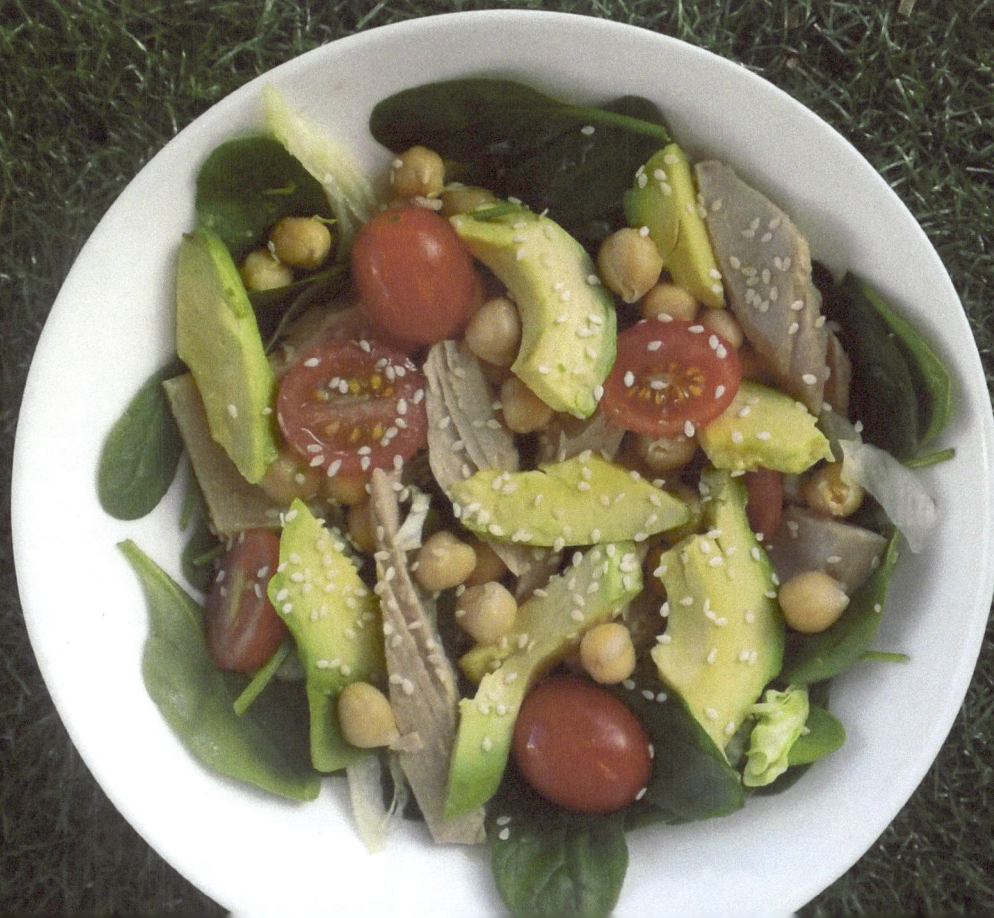

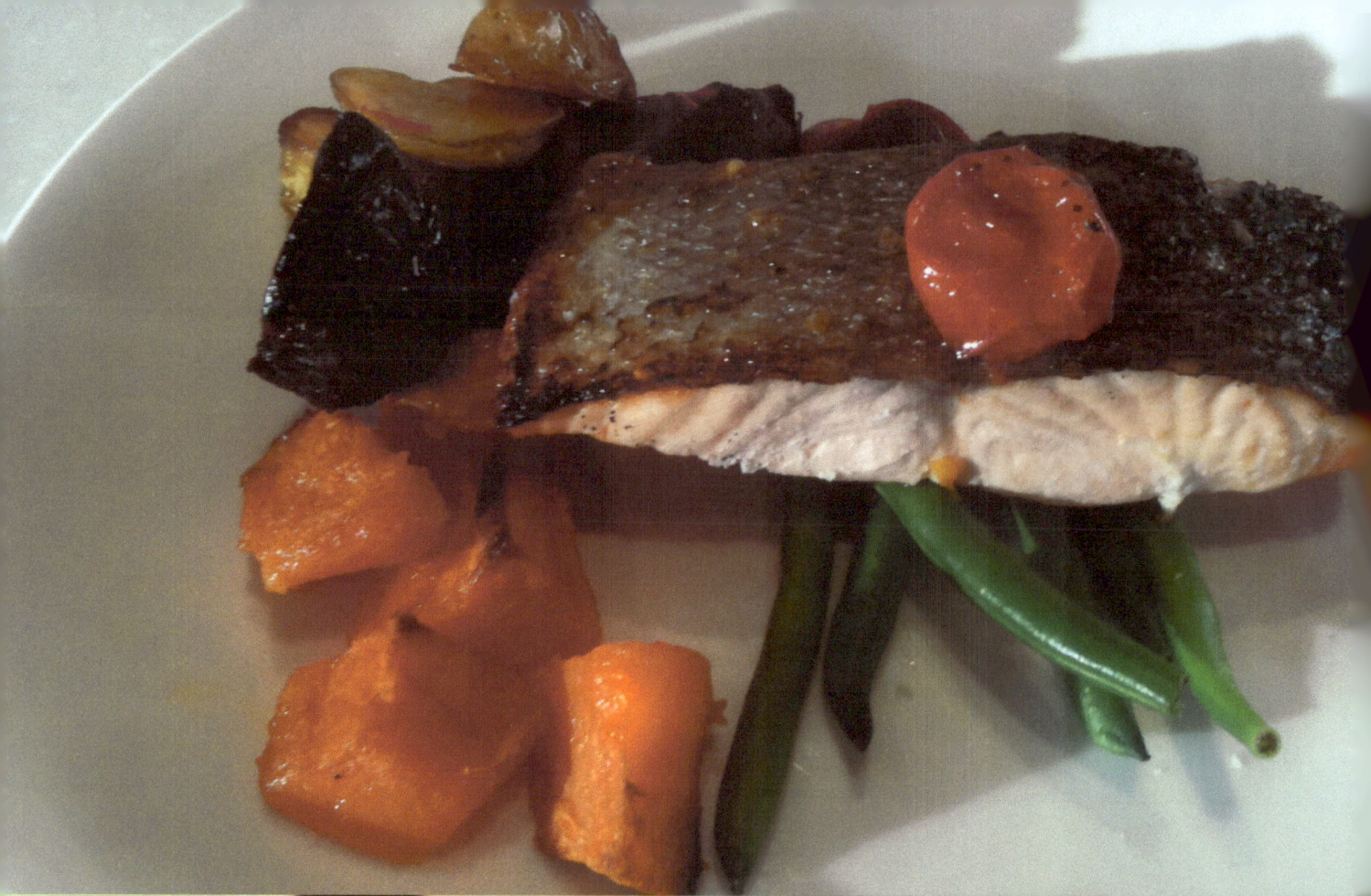

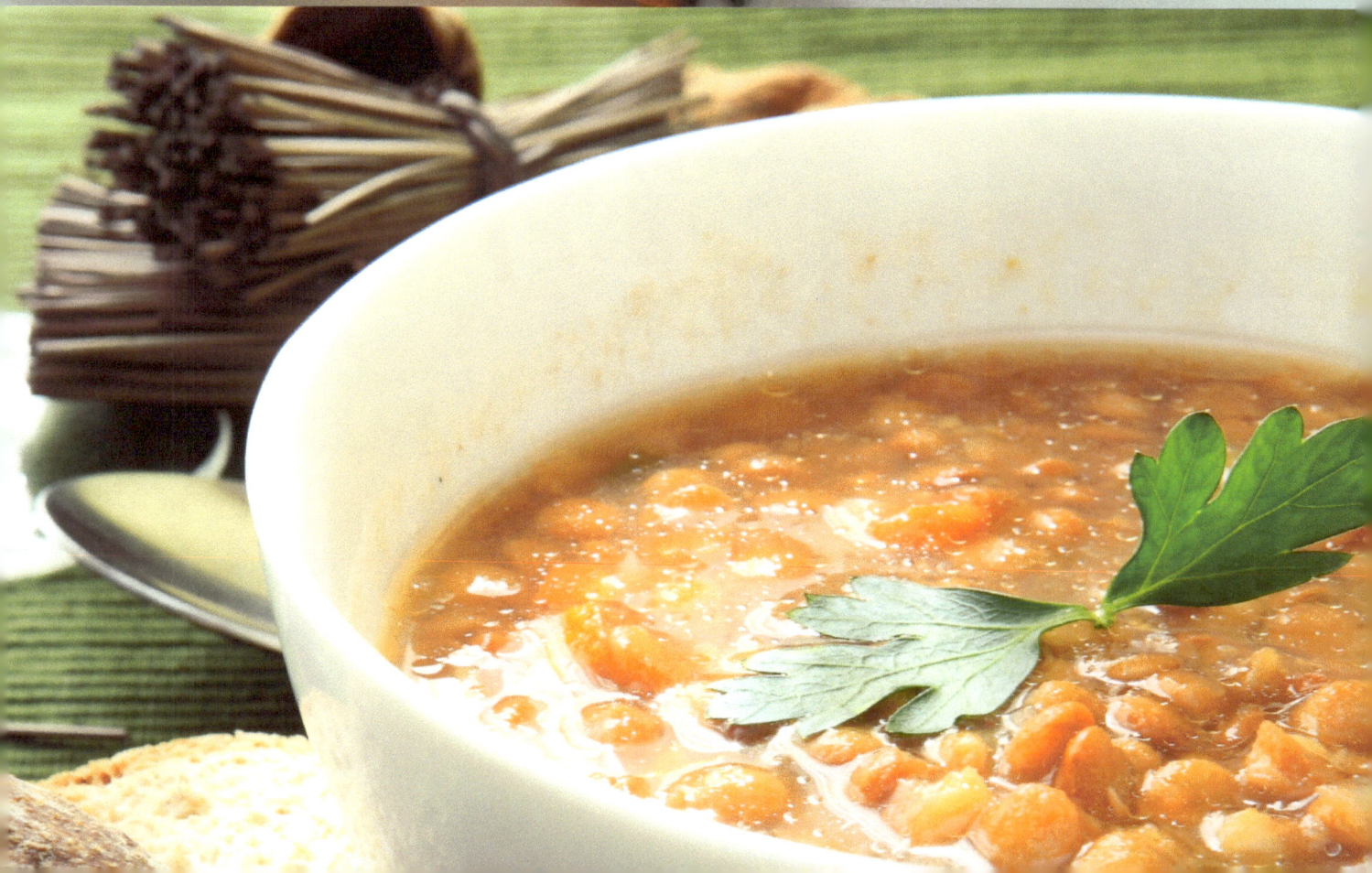

Dinner

Salmon Steak with Roasted Vegetables and Blanched Beans
Serves 2

2 salmon fillets
½ sweet potato, diced
8 shallots or small onions
Handful of green beans
8 cherry or Roma tomatoes

Pre-heat oven to 180 degrees Celsius. Parboil sweet potato and drain. Place in a greased oven tray along with shallots and tomatoes. Bake for 20 minutes.

Heat an oven-proof frypan and add a spray of oil. Place salmon skin down on hot pan and cook for 2-3 minutes on each side. Place salmon in the oven alongside vegetables and bake for a further 5-10 minutes (5 for rare, 10 for medium).

Blanch green beans for 2-3 minutes and serve with salmon and roasted vegetables.

TIP

Cook a little extra salmon and roast vegetables and use it as the base for a delicious salad the next day. For example, add lettuce leaves, avocado and red capsicum.

Red Lentil and Vegetable Soup
Serves 4

1 tablespoon olive oil
1 brown onion, finely chopped
2 cloves garlic, crushed
2 carrots, peeled and diced
2 zucchini, diced
2 sticks celery, diced
1 red capsicum, diced
400g can diced tomatoes
2 cups water
2 cups salt-reduced vegetable stock
375g packet red lentils, rinsed and drained
2 slices of pancetta or ham (optional)

Heat the oil in a large saucepan over a medium heat. Sauté onion and garlic, then add carrots, zucchini, celery and capsicum. Cook for around 10 minutes before adding tomatoes, water, stock, red lentils and pancetta. Bring to the boil before reducing heat to medium-low. Simmer for around 30 minutes, or until lentils are cooked.

Season with freshly ground black pepper and sea salt then serve.

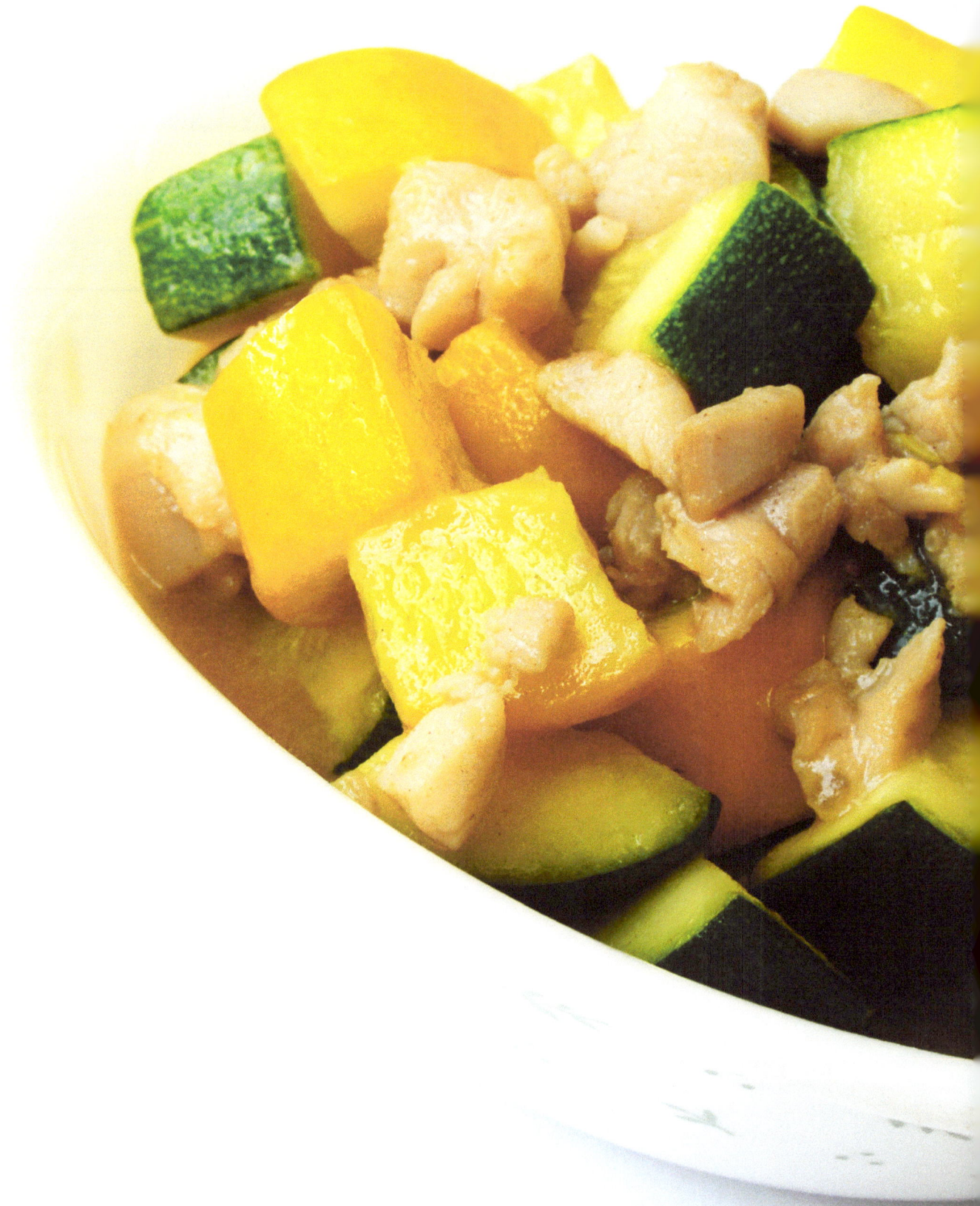

Chicken Stir Fry
Serves 2

300g chicken, diced
1 small onion, diced
2 cloves garlic, crushed,
1 tsp grated ginger
300g mixed vegetables, diced,
2 tbsp tamari (preferably the wheat-free version) or liquid stock
2 tsp sesame seeds
Handful of fresh coriander leaves

Spray oil in wok or fry pan. When heated, add onion, garlic and chicken and stir until browned. Add the rest of the vegetables and cook for 2-3 minutes. Add the tamari or liquid stock and sesame seeds and stir for a further minute.

Mix it up by changing the ingredients:
Protein: pork, beef, lamb or seafood or firm tofu.
Herbs and flavours: lemongrass, parsley, chilli flakes, curry powder
Nuts and seeds: cashew nuts, pine nuts or pumpkin kernels
Vegetables: broccoli, bok choy, red capsicum, asparagus, zucchini, broccolini, baby corn, pumpkin, sweet potato, green beans, spring onion, mushrooms, snow peas, red chillies, etc!

TIP: Cooking meat to perfection

Cook meat, such as steak, chicken or fish, on high temperature on the stove for a few minutes, turn over and place in the oven to finish it off. The oven prevents the moisture from escaping and you will never have to endure dry chicken again! That's how restaurant chefs prepare their meat and most of their vegetables.

Simple vegetable curry
Serves 4

Cooking oil spray
1 medium onion, diced
1 clove garlic, crushed
2 tbsp mild curry powder
2 tbsp rice flour
3 cups vegetable stock
2 carrots, sliced
200g sweet potato or coliban potatoes, diced
1 red capsicum, diced
1 cup peas (frozen)
Steamed rice to serve

1. Spray a large saucepan with oil and heat to medium. Add onion and garlic and cook for 1 minute, stirring. Add curry powder and flour. Add stock and heat till simmering.

2. Add carrots, potatoes and capsicum and simmer for 10 minutes or till potatoes are tender. Stir in peas and cook for further 5 minutes. Serve with steamed basmati or brown rice.

Snacks on the Run

Most of us are out and about during the day, so make sure you don't get too hungry by being prepared with some simple snacks. Put an ice pack in your snack pack or small freezer bag to keep things cool.

- Vegetable strips – carrot, celery, capsicum, zucchini
- Avocado, tzatziki, hummus or mashed roast beetroot, sweet potato or cannellini beans
- Boiled eggs
- Cherry tomatoes
- Green beans
- Soup in a thermos
- Cold meats – turkey, ham off the bone
- Canned fish, such as salmon, sardines or tuna
- Canned beans or corn
- Avocado on corn thins or rice cakes, or wrapped in lettuce leaves
- Fruit – whole or cut it up if it's easier to eat when travelling
- Yoghurt – perhaps frozen
- Almond or cashew butter spreads
- Corn thins or rice cakes
- Peanut butter on celery sticks
- Nuts – almonds, cashews, walnuts, Brazil, macadamias etc.
- Protein shake – maximum of 1 serve a day – after weight training or if no other snack available. Better alternative than nothing or a chocolate bar!

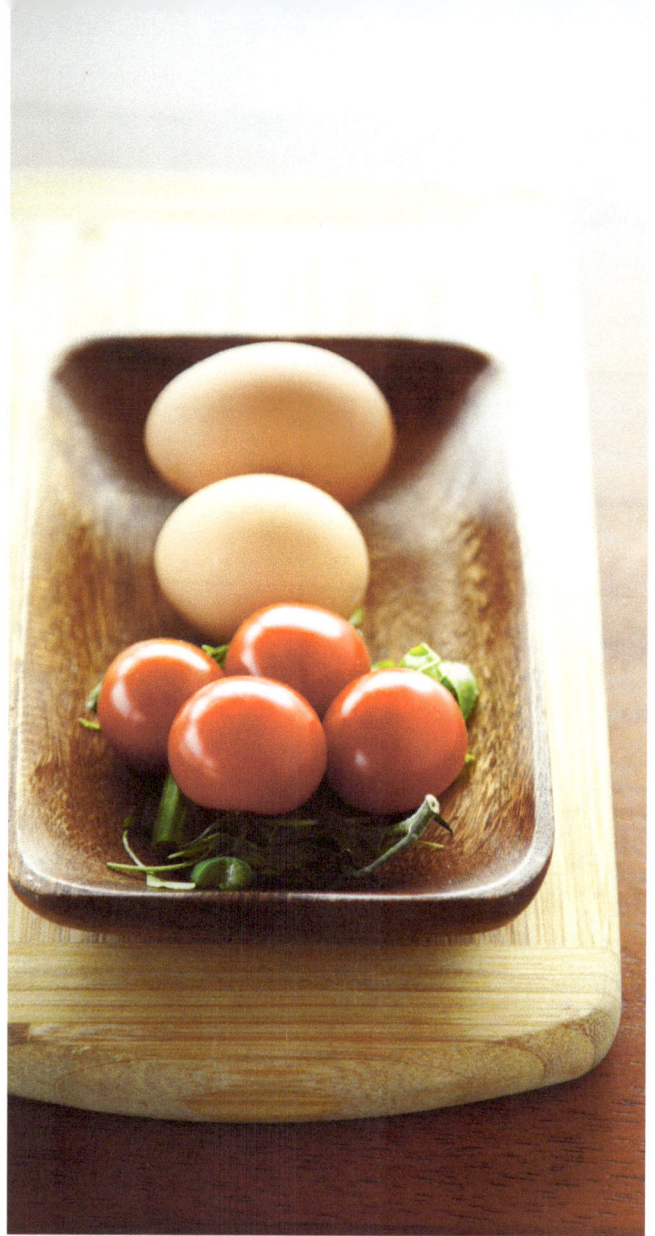

Snack Pack for travelling

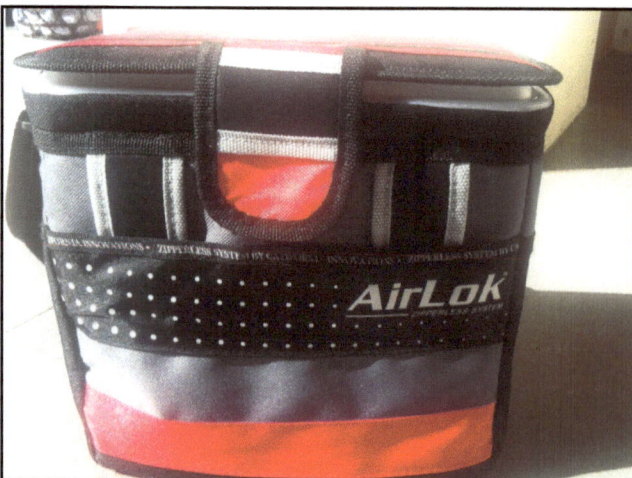

Sample contents of Snack Pack

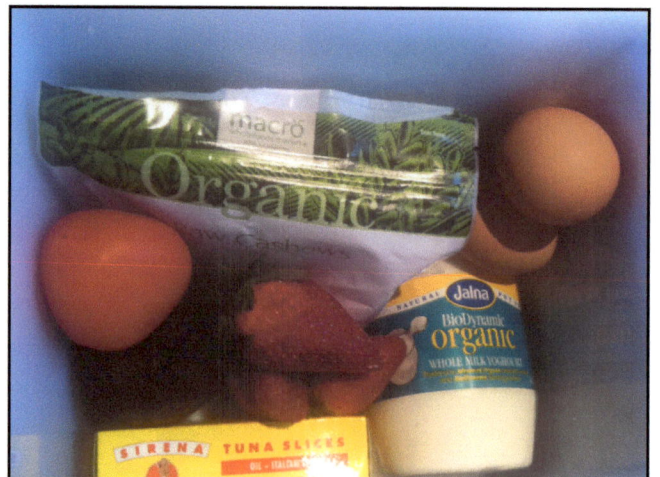

Action

Mind…

What are you prepared to do to get the BEST results? What actions can you take NOW to make some real changes to the way you eat? Write down the changes you can make. You might also like to add them to your list of goals, noting how you will implement them into your daily life. For example, think about the amount of added sugar and nutrient-poor carbohydrates in your diet. What and how much are you willing to eliminate or substitute?

1. _____

2. _____

3. _____

Food…

Start eating the right types of fats, carbohydrates and proteins. Keep it simple and start with:

- Carbohydrates: 40%
- Proteins: 35%
- Fats: 25%
- Change the quality of your carbohydrates. Perhaps buy your fruit and vegetables from local producers and your bread from a baker who values health. Replace poor quality snack foods with dips and grain biscuits, plain pop-corn for the kids and a little dark chocolate for yourself!
- Include the healthy fats in each meal and drop the polyunsaturated oils and trans fats.
- Ensure your protein intake is adequate. Begin by writing out a daily meal planner to ensure you have a good ratio on your plate.
- Drink up! Water not only suppresses the appetite; it rehydrates every cell of your body. It also helps you beat tiredness and improves your muscular strength and metabolism. Drinking water also decreases fat absorption and improves digestion. Drink filtered water and add fresh lemon for a gentle detox and to help clear your digestive tract. Aim for 1.5 to 3 litres of filtered water daily, depending on your weight, the weather and exercise levels. You can mix it up with herbal teas.

Body…

Fuel yourself with living carbohydrates, healthy fats and lean protein most of the time, from now on. Notice how you feel when you eat the right foods – less bloated, more energy, better moods, etc. You will also notice fat loss if you stick to the plan.

Little reminders

1. Refine your food
2. Remove any irritating foods
3. Think quality, not quantity
4. Eat more fresh, uncooked and organic foods, preferably locally-grown
5. Limit or eliminate refined carbohydrates, processed foods, sugar and artificial sweeteners
6. Eat between 3-4pm
7. Chew your food until it's a puree
8. Eat less salt, drink more water

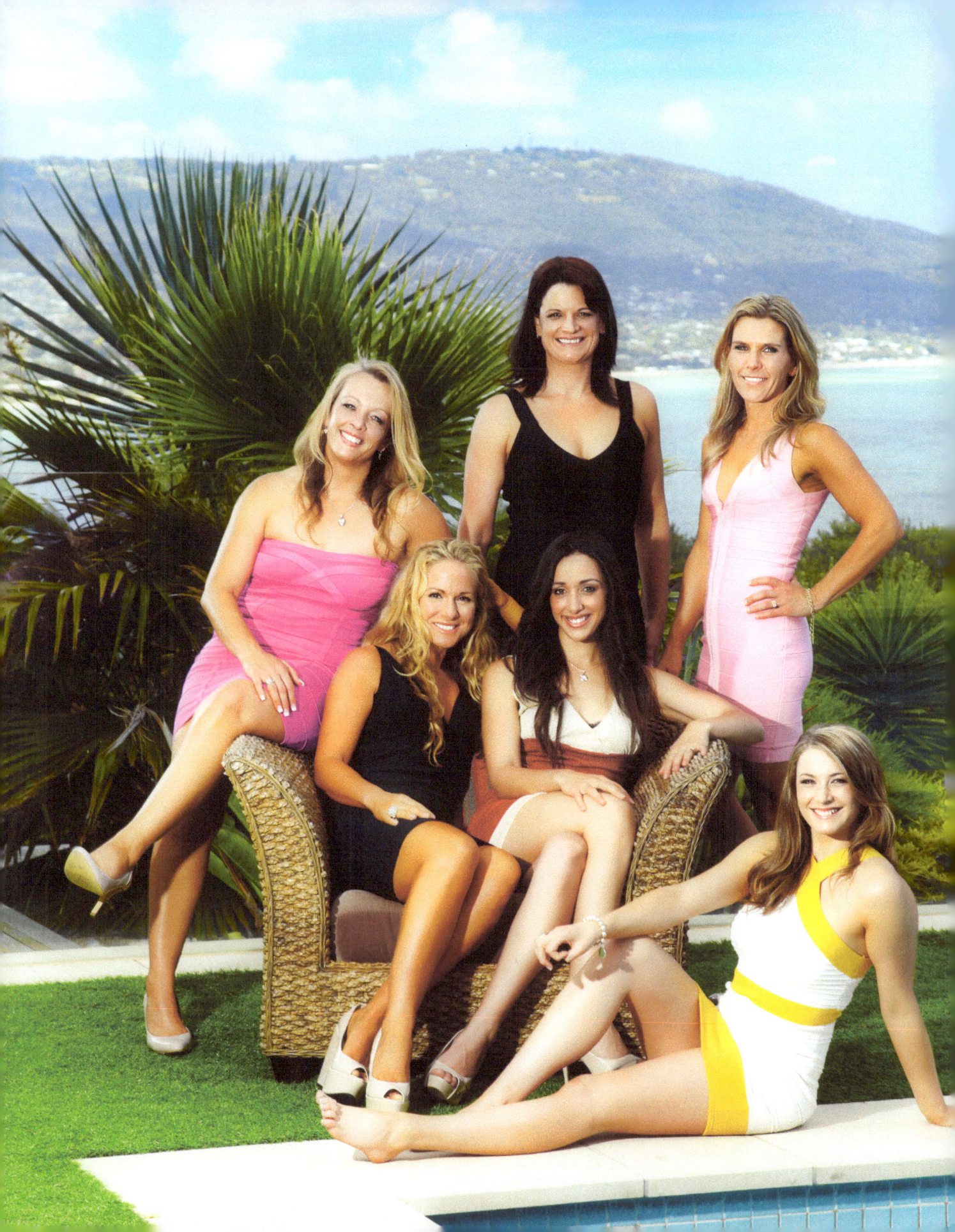

Exercise That Works

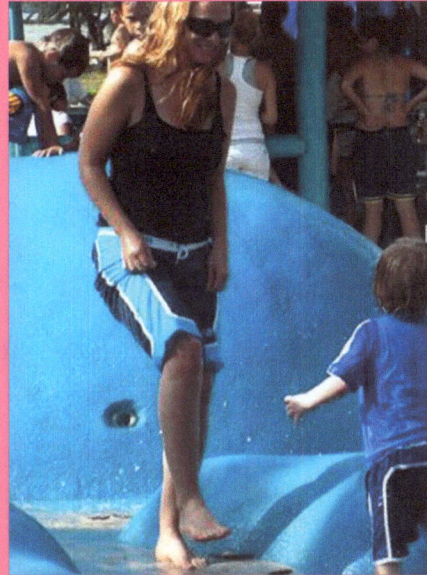
Before: 75kg

"Movement is a medicine for creating change in a person's physical, emotional and mental states"

-Carol Welch

JEN'S STORY

Jen, 39, mother of two, fitness instructor and sales executive

I can't believe I LOVE exercising now after hating it my whole life...

When she was three, Jen's mother emigrated from the United States to Australia, and Jen was introduced to her new dad and three new sisters. With time, Jen settled in to her new life. However, her asthma and allergies made it difficult to join in with the regular pool activities, running around and organised sports. And this, combined with rivalry amongst her new sisters, left Jen feeling second best in any competitive sporting environment. So she avoided competitive sports altogether for fear of always coming last. There was also little encouragement to improve her skills in the physical arena, so over time, she grew to believe she wasn't any good at sport and avoided most physical activity.

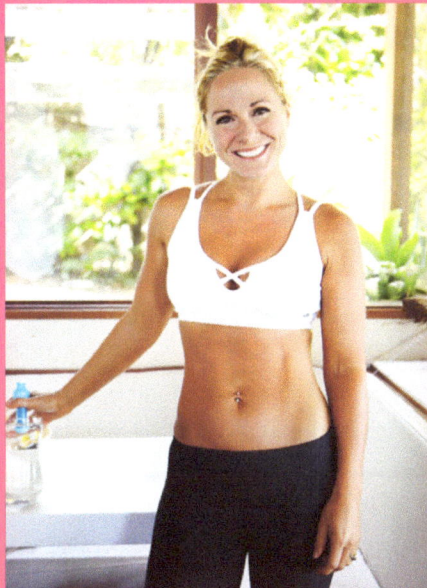
After: 56kg

It wasn't until she was an adult and left work to have her two children that Jen began to reflect on her own health. She was tired of her 'fat clothes' and how she felt about her body. Jen wanted to start feeling good about herself and not tired all the time. She decided it was time to change her life before it passed her by.

Jen had heard time and time again how great exercise made her friends feel, so she started thinking there must be SOME activities she would enjoy. So she put aside her beliefs and negative thoughts on exercise and joined the gym that some of her friends went to. She didn't like it much, but eventually found a couple of classes she enjoyed and slowly but surely, her fitness and confidence grew. She started to realise exercise wasn't as bad as she had imagined!

Jen completed a nutrition course as well, and armed with everything she needed, threw herself into her exercise and improved eating patterns. Within six months, she lost 19kg and 55cm from her body measurements!

Her body fat levels hit an all-time low and she felt and looked like a million dollars. Jen decided to become a fitness instructor and personal trainer so she could help others enjoy their exercise and achieve their goals. As a woman who had 'been there', she understood the feelings of reluctance women faced in relation to exercise. She looked amazing and was a great role model for other women.

I asked Jen some questions about her journey

What was the turning point for you? And how did you get started?

"I had just had enough. Enough of feeling tired, fat, moody and negative. And I thought if I didn't make an effort now, I was going to feel worse in another ten years. I had a friend ten years older than me who looked and felt fantastic, thanks to her exercise and eating habits. It made me realise how differently I could be living my life. After the birth of my second child, I followed her lead and she introduced me to the world of fitness."

JEN'S STATS		
	BEFORE	**AFTER**
Weight:	75kg	56kg
Dress Size:	12-14	8
Time from fat to fab: 6 months		
Key to success: Finding exercise I enjoy doing		

How did you make the transformation from loathing to loving exercise?

"I started to think about all the exercise options available to me - individual and team sports as well as the gym. I thought my local gym was a good place to start as there was a lot of variety under the one roof, and they also had child care, which meant I could exercise whenever it suited me. I managed to find a couple of classes that sounded vaguely interesting, but must say I didn't enjoy the first session. I was very self-conscious and my fitness was so poor it was bloody hard work! However, the instructor was very understanding and reminded me that new people start every day. This helped me through the first session!

I think the real turning point was after my third session, when I had gained a little confidence, as well as coordination. And that's really all it took to get me on the path to really loving exercise and all that it has to offer - I was off and running! The exercise highs gave me energy and great moods and I started to feel really fit. This was a great motivator!

I was really enjoying the cycle class and boxing circuit and this served as a good foundation for learning as well as improving my fitness and strength. I also enlisted the help of a fitness instructor and had a program written for resistance training. After a few weeks, I had learnt a lot and was surprised by how quickly my strength developed. It was at this point that I realised I was LOVING it! And all it took was some initial courage and persistence through the first few sessions."

What has been your most difficult challenge with exercise? How did you keep on track?

"I found the early morning starts hard and occasionally felt like pressing snooze on the alarm. Instead, I thought about how I would feel once I started my workout, when all the happy hormones kicked in, and this got me out of bed. I also reminded myself of the old days – constant fatigue, ill health and sluggishness of the mind and body – and I was off and racing."

What advice do you have for women who don't enjoy exercising?

"If exercise has not been a big part of your life and you're just getting started, it will be a challenge; but remember you are not alone! I thought I hated all forms of exercise before I started, but it turned out it was just fear of the unknown. I didn't realise just how fantastic it would make me feel - and look.

We all go through the mental adjustment of getting started, so just take one day at a time. Take that first step and try some different activities. You will start to feel great very soon and actually look forward to your next session! Your body will adapt to the exercise and you can guide it in the direction you want, which is pretty exciting! So don't let your mind hijack your potential for a fit, strong body.

Most importantly, find something that you enjoy doing! I guess this is where a gym can be so useful. It's a good place to get professional advice, a wide variety of classes and be surrounded by people with common goals.

Set some tangible goals to work towards. At the beginning, these goals will give you a purpose for improving your fitness. It might be to participate in a 5km walk in two months, or be fit enough to join a sporting club. Seek out a committed training partner who will keep you accountable. You will enjoy your exercise much more and you can help and encourage each other. Once you have achieved your goals, adjust them and incorporate something new and exciting to keep you motivated."

What is your weekly exercise program?

"I keep it varied, which is a key element. Otherwise my body tends to get used to the same activity and results slow down. Every week, I complete two weight training sessions, one circuit session and perhaps a walk. I always vary the intensity with all forms of training. When I go walking with a friend, we vary it by going to the beach, the park or walk up hills or along the river track. We call this our 'mental heath' time when we are away from the kids and work. It's so therapeutic to be out in nature, so try it!"

What advice do you have to help prevent women getting bored with their exercise?

"Mix it up! Take your kids to the park while boot camp is on, so you can check out some new ideas and try them for yourself. Ask an instructor or trainer for tips if you need to. Some of the most fun, effective and creative workouts can happen outside of a gym, with a bench and a track. You will be amazed by what you can do with no equipment. Train with a fit friend or ask around to find a training partner. You can learn new ideas and motivate each other. You could also try different classes or join a sports team. And don't forget to set a few goals to give your training more purpose"

What keeps you on a healthy track?

"I think back to my life in my 20s, when I was partying hard, eating badly and really unhealthy. Even then, I knew I could do better for myself. I never realised how great it would feel once I changed my habits. I still enjoy a few wines occasionally, and that's OK, but I never want to return to that lethargic, overweight person. I spent too long feeling unhappy with how I looked. Now I feel great all the time and love the new body I have - I could never give that up. Now I know it's so much easier to maintain a good body once you have it, so I'll never let it go again!"

Exercise: Loving it and Losing Weight

When I ask women: "Why do you exercise?" the answer is almost always the same: "To get fit and lose weight." And usually they *do* improve their fitness, but many women never lose the weight and sometimes gain even more. Why? I think there are three main reasons.

1. They view exercise in a negative light, as punishment, almost, for needing to lose weight. Exercise becomes a chore which must be completed.

2. They don't improve their food intake. In some cases their diet gets worse through rewards or compensatory eating.

3. They do the wrong type of exercise in the belief that more exercise is always better.

Jen's Hot Tips

- Include interval training – it's short, interesting and effective.

- Surround yourself with like minded women who enjoy exercise, sport and good health.

- Establish a weekly and monthly schedule, with a partner if possible, and stick to your activity or exercise sessions like you do other appointments.

- Think about how you could change your routine to fit in exercise right now.

- Imagine you are living someone else's life, perhaps an athlete or someone you aspire to be, and mentally put your face on that person! With effort and determination it will soon be YOU.

Changing your mind

Your body loves it when you're active and your mind can love it too.

If you hate exercise or use it as punishment in an attempt to lose the fat, change how you think about it by finding some activities you actually enjoy.

Being active through sport, an exercise session, or simply playing at the park with the kids is great for both your mind and your body.

- Think how it will make you feel….

  You will have more vitality, improved confidence and better moods. You will feel happy and motivated, energised, yet calm. Exercise will give you focus, a positive state of mind and the patience to manage the kids or a difficult situation in the workplace. It will give you the energy and clarity of mind to be really productive in your day. Have you noticed that people who exercise often have these traits? You too can be free of the afternoon slump, unexplainable bad moods or brain fog, forever.

- Think about what it will do for your body…

You will develop good muscle tone, lose fat, improve your strength, flexibility and functionality, prevent disease, live longer and age more slowly. You will have the strength and fitness needed to run and play football with the kids and of course the muscle tone you want to see in the mirror! The body is amazingly adaptable to any challenge you give it – even if you haven't exercised in years.

Focus on how great exercise is for your mind and body. Set your mind on what you want. For example, imagine the new lean and fit body you want, rather than getting rid of the body you don't want. The greatest success with fat loss actually comes to women who focus on positives, such as their fitness goals and how great they feel, rather than on how overweight they think they are. The by-product of increased fitness WILL be fat loss. All the women in this book did just that. Channel your energy in a positive direction for results. The quality of your life will improve forever.

Compensation, rewards, guilt and more exercise…

Sometimes exercise promotes overeating or poor food choices. After exercise, do you eat more or eat unhealthy food as a reward? Do you find that you want to move less for the rest of the day after you have exercised?

A 2008 study published in the International Journal of Obesity found that when the 538 subjects exercised, they ate an average of 100 calories *more* than they had just burned. This may be true for many of us.

Perhaps the following scenario sounds familiar:
A woman completes a workout on the cardio equipment at the gym for an hour in the morning, and catches up for a coffee with a friend afterwards. By the time she has two coffees and says goodbye, she is starving. She eats a large sandwich, but is still hungry and is craving something sweet. She figures she has exercised hard, so she deserves a muffin. When she gets home, she is exhausted and spends the rest of the day resting! The next day, she feels guilty about the muffin and 'punishes' herself on the treadmill for an hour… and the cycle continues.

Many women report various versions of this scenario. Having the right strategies in place can get you off this rollercoaster.

You already have the tools to prepare nutritious meals. Combine this with knowledge on how to match your food intake to the requirements of your physically active body, and all the pieces will come together for great results. Learning how to avoid eating as a reward for exercise, or overeating due to excessive hunger, will have you feeling great all day.

Fuelling for Exercise

So many women don't think about how they eat before and after exercising.

Over the past 20 years, I have discovered that what you eat **just prior and immediately after** any type of exercise is a key element to fitness, health and fat loss.

It is at this time the body will benefit the most from the 'fuel' you provide it. Eating correctly will affect your performance while exercising, prevent muscle breakdown, determine how well you recover from exercise, and even affect the quantity and quality of the food you eat for the rest of the day. You will also find your energy levels will be improved if you fuel well over the next couple of days. Eating well will keep your cortisol levels in check, which prevents stress on the body, weight gain *and* makes you feel good.

Your body needs to be fed **well** before it is put to the test and refuelled once you have finished. It makes sense and is the key to feeling good and losing weight.

Before Exercise

Ideally, eat a meal around three hours before any strength training session to allow adequate time to digest the meal. The closer to a workout food is eaten, the smaller the meal or snack should be. If there is only two hours before you plan to exercise, just have a light meal. If you have an hour or so before training and you need to fuel, try a protein smoothie or vegetable juice.

- It's best to listen to your body and eat only as much as you feel you can properly digest before exercising.
- Avoid high fat, high fibre foods that can't be digested quickly, and also gaseous foods such as beans, to reduce the risk of stomach discomfort.
-
- Drink around half a litre of water in the hours before a workout - or the evening before, if it is an early morning session - to ensure the body is properly hydrated.

During Exercise

The fluids or fuel you require during exercise usually depend on the type and duration of the activity. If you are doing cardio or weight training for up to an hour, 100 to 200ml of water for every 15 to 30 minutes of exercise is ideal.

If you are exercising at a high intensity for over an hour (especially if it's hot), you might consider sipping a sports drink or taking an electrolyte gel or banana with you to replace the simple carbohydrates and electrolytes you have lost.

NOTE: Consult with a trainer or coach if you think this may apply to you.

After Exercise

Rehydration after your workout is essential. To find out how much you need to drink, try weighing yourself before and after your workout. Any weight lost will be water, so drink one to two cups of water for each 500g lost.

How you eat after exercising determines your energy levels and recovery for the day AND your next work out! Your window of opportunity to most effectively re-fuel your body after its efforts is around 30 minutes – so have a snack ready to go. The ideal snack after exercise will depend on the type of exercise you have done.

Weight Training

Eating a snack packed with protein and carbohydrates within half an hour of exercising ensures your body has the fuel when it really needs it to restock glycogen stores, build and repair muscle tissue. One study has pinpointed 20gms as the ideal amount of post-workout protein to maximise muscle repair and growth.

Avoid fructose (including fruit juices) for two hours after training, as it will stop your natural human growth hormone production, which is vital for muscle growth.

"If you're lifting weights and don't consume protein, it's almost counterproductive"
Jeffrey Volek

Cardio Training

As with weight training, consume a carbohydrate and protein snack within half an hour of training, the sooner the better. Concentrate on simple carbohydrates and replacing electrolytes if you have trained hard for over an hour. You will have lost some of these vital minerals when exercising for long durations or in hot conditions. Then eat a balanced meal within an hour or so.

Now let's consider how you can most effectively exercise for a lean, toned body.

BEFORE TRAINING
3 hours before ALL training: protein and carbohydrate-rich meal, limited fats

- Homemade Muesli with yoghurt or milk (see recipe)
- Chicken and Sugar Snap Pea Salad (see recipe)
- Chicken or turkey wrap with lettuce, tomato, avocado and sprouts
- Grilled fish with brown rice and vegetables

Less than 2 hours before ALL training: light snack or meal, low fibre, limited fats

- Very Berry Smoothie (see recipe)
- Fruit salad and yoghurt
- Calamari salad with light dressing

30 min before training: light snack

Weight Training
1 serve of protein
- protein shake (easy to make and quickly used by muscles)
- 2-3 eggs
- tub of yoghurt
- cottage cheese

Cardio Training
1 serve of carbohydrates
- 1 banana, apple or orange
- glass of juice
- rice cakes with tomato
- Avoid simple sugars such as lollies, to prevent blood sugar crashes and energy slumps

AFTER TRAINING
Within 30 minutes: snack

Weight Training
1 serve of protein and carbohydrates
- protein smoothie or protein powder with a banana
- peanut butter or lean meat sandwich
- rice cakes with cheese, chicken or turkey
- baked beans with cheese on top
- eggs on toast/ corn thins

Cardio Training
Carbohydrate-rich snacks
- yoghurt with fruit salad
- glass of fruit/ vegetable juice, fruit smoothie or glass of milk
- oats with milk
- vegetables and hommus
- sports drink (for intense exercise of >1 hour)

Around 1 hour after ALL training:
protein and carbohydrate-rich meal, including fats

- baked or grilled fish (150g) and vegetables
- chicken (120g), salad and a jacket potato
- burger – 100g lean mince pattie and salad in wholegrain roll
- ½ - 1 cup steamed rice and stir fry vegetables with almonds
- ham or tuna and salad wrap
- baked beans on toast
- Red Lentil and Vegetable Soup (see recipe) with toast

Balanced Exercise for Health and Fat Loss

Sometimes we need to exercise smarter for more fat loss…..

A common misconception is that the longer you exercise the more calories you will burn and therefore the more fat you will lose. However, it doesn't always work that way.

Although Australians spend an estimated $735 million a year on club memberships, as well money spent on other exercise, overweight and obesity figures continue to rise. Certainly, regular exercise *can* have an impact on our weight, but if most of us are still overweight what are we doing wrong?

Doing lots of classes at the gym or walking for hours on the treadmill is not the answer to long-term fat loss. If you have embarked on a gruelling exercise program with NO results in the fat loss department; it may be time to ask yourself why.

Some recent studies have found that doing just *cardio* exercise does not lead to significant fat loss. Does this suggest that many of us are doing the *wrong type* of exercise and for too long if our main objective is weight loss?

Cardio exercise of more than an hour typically does not involve sufficient intensity to effectively shed excess fat and build muscle. Of course you burn calories, but you won't improve your body composition, you may be breaking down your muscle stores and you're more prone to injuries.

It *is* actually possible to achieve better results with less work as long as it is the right type of exercise. If you know how to train smarter, rather than harder, you will lose the fat faster.

It's not just about the amount of time you allocate to either weight training or cardio exercise – *longer is not necessarily better*. The type, method and intensity of all the exercise you do are key elements to your success.

If your main objective is to lose the fat and gain lean muscle in order to get the trim, toned body you want, you need to get the right balance of cardio and weight training, with the scales tipped in favour of weight training.

Liz is the perfect example. She trained for over an hour 6 days a week – and she trained HARD. She did long bike rides, classes and some weights. However, she was still 100kg, with no change on the scales in sight. As soon as she began to eat well and train for shorter time periods and less frequently she began to lose weight.

Weight training is the only way to prevent muscle loss and build muscle tissue. By improving your muscle mass, your body will be more toned and your resting metabolism will be increased. This means you will burn a lot more energy than someone who has less muscle mass.

Research studies have shown that if we increase our lean muscle mass by 1.4kg we also increase our resting metabolism by 7%. Research also revealed that this can be achieved with a basic weight training program lasting just 25 minutes, followed three times a week, for a total of 8 weeks!

Cardio is your weapon to get fit and burn some calories, but it won't help you build muscle; rather it promotes muscles breakdown.

Initially, work towards completing three weight training sessions and two cardio sessions a week to be on track for some great results. Once you have achieved your ideal body, you may even be able to drop it back to two weight training sessions and two short cardio sessions for maintenance. This could mean training for a total of just 2-3 hours a week!

Weight Training

From the age of around 20, you lose more than 200 grams of muscle each year if you are inactive. By 40 years of age, without weight training, your body fat levels will be sky high and 'tuck shop arms' are pretty much a certainty.

Weight training doesn't have to mean looking like a body builder. Most of us simply want to change the ratio of muscle to fat in order to look toned and lean. A sensible weight training program along with good eating can give you the body and strength of someone years younger.

Let's look at the magical health benefits of resistance or weight training. These should give you enough reasons to get you pumping a little iron!

- Reduced insulin levels in the blood (less blood sugar to store as fat)

- Improved strength and muscle mass

- Increased metabolic rate

- Reduced cortisol levels, which promotes fat loss

- Increased human growth hormone levels – vital for strength, fat loss and longevity

- Improved bone density – lowering the risk of osteoporosis

- Improved functioning of the body – the ability to climb stairs and lift heavy items

- Reduced body fat and incidence of obesity

- Improved balance

- Reduced resting blood pressure

- Improved glucose metabolism – assisting in the prevention of adult onset diabetes

- Improved cholesterol levels

- Improved appearance and self-confidence

- Improved sleep

- Decreased risk or rate of depression

- Reduced back pain, arthritic pain and improved mobility

Muscle tissue has a much higher metabolic rate than fat tissue and burns almost three times the amount of calories. So once you have developed good muscle mass, your muscles themselves are an effective fat loss weapon - even while you are at rest.

There is an impressive 'after burn effect' as a result of weight training. The amount of calories burnt *after* you exercise is significant. Studies have found that the after burn effect of weight training is highly effective in raising metabolic rates, and thus, burning calories. This is the vital link between exercise and fat loss.

This effect is increased with bursts of intense weight training rather than training at a slower rate. One study, published in the *European Journal of Applied Physiology* in 2011, showed that subjects used an extra 100 calories a day for three days when they did EITHER one or three sets of intense resistance training. So one set is just as effective – I like the sound of that!

Working at a higher intensity also increases the effects. A 2011 study (Knab et al) showed that subjects who cycled at a high intensity burned an additional 37% more calories *after the day after* the workout. So a single high-intensity session burns a lot of extra energy. A low-intensity session will basically just burn calories during the activity.

Cardiovascular Exercise

Cardiovascular exercise (or aerobic training) elevates your heart rate for an extended period of time. It will improve your heart strength and lung health, allow you to perform your everyday activities with ease, release hormones for great moods, help you relax and reduce the risk of many diseases.

Walking, swimming, dancing, cycling and yoga are cardio activities which you can do at any intensity. In combination with a weight training program, cardio exercise will accelerate the fat burning process. It should not be used as a substitute for weight training, as *it does not permanently increase your metabolism or have the ability to re-shape your body.*

Cardiovascular exercise is most effective for fat loss when it is performed intensely, for shorter periods of between 20-45 minutes. So 20 minutes, twice a week for cardio can be enough!

With high intensity cardio training, your fitness level will improve at a much faster rate and there is less wear and tear on the body, as the activity is over much sooner. You can train harder without stressing the body as much and it can also be a much more enjoyable way to exercise. Most importantly, it will give you more effective fat loss results.

Real Woman Workouts

It's time for you to get moving! Decide whether you will begin at Level 1 or 2, depending on your current fitness level.

REAL WOMAN WORKOUT – Level 1

If you are currently doing no exercise, use a blank weekly calendar to list some bite sized goals. For example, on Monday, Wednesday and Friday introduce a 15 minute walk before or after work or at lunchtime. Then increase the time spent walking to 20, then 30 minutes. Once this is a regular activity over three weeks, you will have succeeded at establishing a habit. This means you are now *used to* setting aside the time to exercise and will have gained some fitness along the way. You will then be ready to introduce some resistance or weight training.

You may like to exercise outside, in your home, at a sporting club or in a gym. You could incorporate walking up and down the stairs, jogging on the spot, bike riding with the kids, or doing laps in the pool. Work out what you enjoy and write out your weekly program, like this:

Getting Started

WEEK 1

20 minute session including:

- Walk (flat ground)

- Home workout

- Stair climbing

- Walk (beach on soft sand or hills)

WEEK 2

30 minute session including:

- Long walk (flat ground)

- Home workout

- Stair climb

- Pilates or yoga session

WEEK 3

Increase the intensity of each session

If you feel ready to hit the gym, join up and follow the advice of the staff. They will take you through the training programs.

If you cannot access a gym or would prefer to train at home, try the following basic program. It is a combination of interval training and resistance work, which will establish a strong foundation of fitness.

To achieve great results, it's best to include some weights later on.

Home Workout

Warm up before each session with a 5-10 minute walk or bike ride, then allow between 20 minutes (Week 1 and 2) and 40 minutes (Weeks 3 and 4) to complete this workout.

Exercise

Skip or jog on spot	Keep tummy in, shoulders neutral.
Push Ups	On knees initially, lower body weight to floor using chest muscles. Contract stomach muscles gently throughout the movement.
Squats	Imagine you are about to sit on a chair. Keep knees behind toes, bend backwards and down from the hips. Start movement from the hips. Buttocks move outwards and downwards with your back straight, chest up. Lift arms up in front as you squat.
Elbow plank	Lie on a mat on your front, lift body weight and support on forearms and toes. Abdominal muscles tight, body in a straight line – no sagging in the lower back. If you need to take the pressure off your lower, lift hips slightly.
Step ups	Step up onto a step or low bench. Step down using the opposite foot first. Focus on using buttocks and thigh muscles.
Dips	Sit on the edge of a low bench or step. Keep hands in close by side, elbows in, feet out in front. Lower body to floor by bending elbows. Stage 1: feet on floor. Stage 2: heels on floor.
Wall sit	Stand against wall with feet slightly away, and then lower your body so that your thighs are 90 degrees to the ground in a sitting position.
Crunches	Lying on the floor, knees bent with feet on the floor. Contract stomach muscles gently by drawing the navel towards the floor. With arms across your chest, slowly lift your shoulders off the floor then return to starting position.
Stretch Hold for 20 secs each side	Thighs: lift foot and grasp ankle, holding it behind thigh Shoulders: cross arm across your body and use other hand to push forearm towards chest.

WEEK 1 30secs, 10sec rest, repeat x 2

WEEK 2 30 secs, no rest, repeat x 3

WEEK 3/4 45 secs, 15 sec rest, repeat x 4

Repeat this first stage of training for around 4 weeks, or until you feel your body is ready for weight training and Level 2.

Weight Training
Now it's time to introduce some resistance training into your weekly program. Join a gym, even just for a few months to get some expert guidance. Book a session to have a fitness assessment and an introductory program. The instructor will write a personalised program for you and take you through it.

This program will take into consideration your fitness level, any restrictions or injuries and your past weight training experience.

You can also check out the classes at your gym and consider what might suit you to get started. Most gyms have a large range of classes, including cycle, boxing, circuits, 'Pump' (weights to music), as well as cardio-based classes.

Weight Training Tips
Whether you choose the gym or home to work out, it's always good to understand the steps involved in weight training. Learning the correct techniques will condition your joints and build a base of strength and stability. This sets the foundation for some intense – and effective – weight training.

The staff at your gym can give you expert advice on your personal program. Use their expertise to get the most out of your sessions. Here are a few tips to get you thinking about what to do.

Warm Up

Start with a 5-10 minute warm up to increase the blood flow to muscles, so that they are ready to move efficiently and less likely to injure yourself. This can be something as simple as walking or cycling.

Technique

- Enlist the help of a trainer to demonstrate and check your technique.

- On the first set, warm up the muscles you are using by performing a set with light weights.

- Switch on your core gently.

- Concentrate on using the correct muscles and breathe out on the contraction or exertion phase.

Starting Weight

Use trial and error to work out your starting weight. This way, you will be learning how to gauge the appropriate weight needed for each exercise. In the first few sessions, err on the side of caution.

As you progress, select the heaviest weight that allows you to complete your repetitions while still maintaining proper form. If you can complete all your repetitions without struggling to get the last repetition, then the weight is too light. If you have to change your body posture or alter the motion, then the weight is too heavy.

Repetitions

Ensure your muscles are under tension for the whole movement. Each repetition should take 4-6 seconds. Start with 12-15 repetitions and rest for one minute between each set.

Frequency

Perform your weight training program 2-3 times a week. A full-body program is a gentle introduction to weight training, and ideal for conditioning your body.

Duration

The good news is that it only takes 20-30 minutes to promote muscle growth, give your metabolism a big boost and improve your strength. That's the key: working less and getting more out of your workouts for great results.

Weight Stations or Free Weights?

If you are new to weights, use the weight machines at the gym for the first three weeks. Ask a fitness instructor for help to perfect your technique. The weighted cable or hydraulic machines give you the opportunity to learn how an exercise should feel before moving onto free weights, which are slightly more difficult to master. Free weights are the most effective method as your body must control the whole movement, using more muscles and energy as well as core stability. Seek expert advice on the most suitable option for you.

Variety = success

A combination of weight training and cardiovascular exercise is the most effective method to improve fitness and lose fat.

Gather all the information and plan out a suitable weekly routine. To get the right balance of weights and cardio exercise, aim for 2-3 weight sessions and 1-2 cardio sessions.

Weight training will improve your strength and enable your body to build the muscle tissue it needs in order to lose the fat. Cardiovascular activities benefit your health and fitness, as well as increasing the amount of energy used, which is also important for fat loss.

Now that you have the basics, let's move onto some strategies for further success in fitness and leanness of body.

REAL WOMAN WORKOUT - Level 2

With a solid foundation of fitness under your belt, you can now begin to enjoy a wider variety of activities. To really improve your fitness and strength, it's time to increase the intensity and variety.

You can introduce heavier weights and different exercises, as well as train at a higher rate to stimulate change in your body and really progress. Get some advice on plyometrics, pyramid, periodised and interval strength training for variety to improve fitness and prevent boredom!

For example, 'super sets' involve performing two exercises one after the other before resting. Studies have shown enhanced calorie burning during weight training with super sets (Haltom et al 1999). You could try a set of split lunges, followed by a dumbbell shoulder press. Work opposing muscle groups or upper and lower body parts for more compound or whole body movements.

You can keep your weights workout to 30 minutes. This is adequate time to put your muscles through their paces to get results.

Ask the instructor at the gym for a new program which includes a completely new set of exercises for different muscle groups.

Aim for four to five sessions of exercise per week, 3 weight training and 1-2 cardio activities. Schedule your program into your diary or monthly calendar like all your other appointments.

TAKE NOTE: If you miss any training, skip the cardio. You can really get great results from 3 weights sessions of 30 minutes, as long as your food is really clean 90% of the time…Isn't that great news!

WEEK 1
- Boxing class or beach run
- Weight training – circuit
- Skipping and swim
- Weight training - explosive
- Weight training – heavy

WEEK 2
- Pump class
- Stair runs
- Weight training – super sets
- Pilates or yoga
- Weight training

WEEK 3/4 Combine week 1 & 2 with different intensities and type of training.

Cardio sessions (outside of gym classes) only need to be 20-45 minutes long. Record the times and distances of your cardio activities to monitor your progress. Aim to improve times or distances at each session.

Now that you have some ideas on what to do and why, go for it! You will learn more as you progress, through experimentation and the advice of others. Love what you do and your body will love it too.

Action

Mind...

Visualise yourself exercising regularly, living a fit life. Imagine yourself as an aspiring athlete, or someone who loves exercising and sport. The mind is so powerful, so give it the right thoughts to bring about change. Perhaps think of someone you know like this, and ask them how they fit everything into their lives. Emulate their methods, rather than reinventing the wheel.

Change your focus from losing weight to getting fit and enjoy the many benefits you receive along the way.

Swap these thoughts:
* "I'm so fat, I hate how I look",

* "It's all too hard",

* "It's not working anyway",

For positive inner-talk:
* "I feel so happy and full of energy for the whole day after exercise."

* "I can do anything I want now that I am stronger and fitter. I can lift anything and run with the kids without feeling out of breath."

* "My body feels great and is more toned than ever before".

*Focus on what you WANT to achieve,
not on what you DON'T want*

Body...

If you regularly do the same type of exercise, your body becomes conditioned to that activity and will perform it with the least amount of exertion and energy. You need to stimulate and stress your muscles and cardiovascular system for growth and improvement. Your body will resist change – so force it into action with variety.

Varying your work outs will give you great results. Change your routine and leave your comfort zone to encourage your body to lose fat. It also keeps things more interesting and motivating. This requires that you think about your activities and do some planning – you won't accidently reach your goals. Put a strategic plan in place, rather than just doing what you always do – and vary every session in some way. If you want to see regular changes and progress with your body, change any of the following:

* Duration or distance

* Intensity

* Environment

* Type of activity or equipment

* Number of repetitions or sets

* Recovery time and method

For example, vary the intensity of your runs to include hills or sprint work. Your fitness will improve dramatically and your flat runs will be a lot easier and faster. If you are weight training, lift heavy weights to fatigue session one, use lighter weights at a faster rate in session two, and complete a different group of exercises in the third session.

Food...

Focus on how you eat around your training. Maximise your results by eating good quality protein and carbohydrates for optimal recovery.

Leaping Hurdles

Before: 60kg

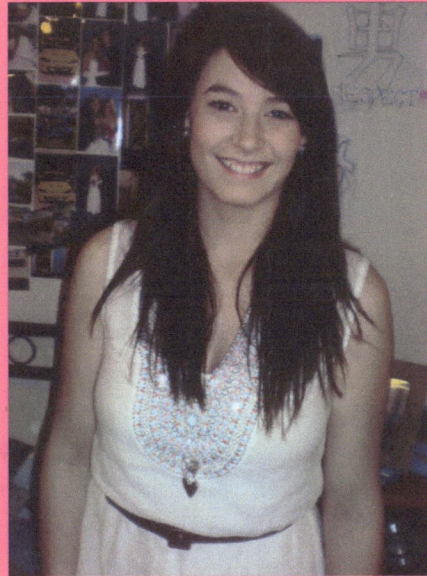

"Accept the challenges so that you can feel the exhilaration of victory"

George S. Patton

JADE'S STORY

Jade, 23, in a relationship, lives with her mum, advertising executive

I felt that exercise brought me closer to my dad – as though he was watching over me. Fitness was something we shared together, so this kept me focussed.

After: 55kg

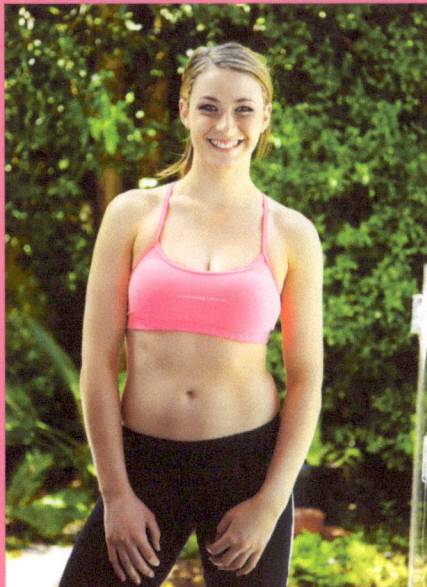

Jade's father Guy was a great athlete in his day, competing for Victoria in athletics and playing football for Hawthorn before retiring to support his family with a 'proper' paying job. When Jade was a young girl, it became apparent to Guy that his daughter was a naturally talented athlete too. Her genes helped, but she also loved sport and thrived on the challenge of competition, so father and daughter exercised together regularly.

Guy could see the enormous potential Jade had as an athlete, so at the age of 11, she began training professionally. With her dad as her coach, Jade took to the training happily and was highly focussed.

Her mum, brother and Nanna were also very supportive throughout her years of growing up. They would regularly watch her compete at the Athletics track and cheer as she continually beat her personal best times.

Her abilities and confidence grew, and by the age of 17 her sights were set on the 2008 Beijing Olympics. She was beating the country's best runners in 1500m races and looked ready to secure her place in the Beijing team.

Then her father was diagnosed with cancer. This put an end to Jade's dream, as her heart just wasn't in it anymore. She gave up training to help her dad in their family business. After a long struggle, Guy succumbed to the disease. Jade was only 19.

With her father gone, Jade fell into a black hole. She grieved deeply and nothing seemed to matter anymore. She stopped exercising at all, and found herself tired, unfit and unmotivated. She just couldn't seem to get going again after losing her coach and mentor.

Jade was fortunate to have a brilliant support network around her. Her mother, brother and in later years, her boyfriend were always there for her. This made her journey a lot easier to manage in the tough times. They have helped her to achieve every goal, every step of the way.

Eventually, Jade came out the other side of her grieving. She realised that not living her own life would not bring her father back. She knew her father wouldn't want her to neglect her health or spend her days feeling sorry for herself. Jade realised that life was short, so she had better make the most of it. She decided that her health and fitness was her number one priority and she wanted to tone up, so she began to change her life.

As an athlete, Jade had always been armed with a strong sense of self-belief and once again, she had a

JADE'S STATS		
	BEFORE	**AFTER**
Weight:	60kg	55kg
Dress Size:	10-12	8
Time from fat to fab: 4 months		
Key to success: Overcoming obstacles with resilience		

vision firmly in mind. Jade had a goal – to exude fitness and health. She wanted to become a personal trainer and look the part, too.

Jade began by improving the quality of the food she was eating, every single day. She had just moved in with her boyfriend and his family and as she learnt more about eating well she excitedly shared her techniques with them. Jade's housemates also achieved some health benefits through her new way of eating. She also began to regain her fitness with some short runs and interval sessions and started to feel good again.

Every day she achieved a little more and over the next six months, she took all the right steps. Of course there were some hurdles along the way. Jade discovered she was gluten intolerant, so she learned what she could about the condition and what she could do to manage it, although it was hard while living under someone else's roof. She also took an overseas trip and had to negotiate her dietary needs while she was away. She worked long hours, leaving little time for exercise or food preparation, and even moved house.

She somehow came to enjoy these challenges to her routine, and went on to become a vision of health.

I asked Jade some questions about her journey

Can you tell us a little about your childhood?
"Growing up, I loved two things dearly – Dad and running. I loved the freedom running gave me and the sense of accomplishment as I got faster and won more competitions. Dad was integral to that, as he saw the

potential in me and provided the encouragement I needed to believe in myself. Dad was a fantastic coach and mentor and I would never have got to Olympic level without him.

When Dad was diagnosed with bowel cancer, I decided that my family was more important than running. It wasn't fair on Dad to be getting up early each morning to train me. So I stopped training and spent all my time with Dad, helping to run our family spring water business. I will never regret that decision, as he is no longer here.

When Dad passed away, I couldn't think about the future at all, let alone set any goals I wanted to accomplish. Losing the two things I cherished, Dad and running, took away all my passion, and I lost interest in everything."

What was the moment you decided to change your body and your health?

"In my months of grieving, I did no exercise and my diet was unhealthy, but I didn't care. It all seemed irrelevant for a while. Then one day about six months later, I looked at myself in the mirror and wondered what I was doing to myself. Dad would not want me to be feeling sorry for myself or neglecting my health and fitness. And with great support from my mum and brother, I got focussed. I bought a treadmill and my adventure began."

How did you begin changing your diet?

"I had some excess weight I could not seem to lose with exercise – so I thought about what and how I was eating. I knew I had to change my eating habits in order to obtain the fit, trim body I wanted. I completed a nutrition course and gained all the knowledge I needed. At the start it was extremely difficult, as I am a chocolate lover like many other women in the world! Also I was hungry all the time, and never understood why, until I learnt I didn't have enough protein in my diet. I was eating too many refined carbohydrates, which explained why I was carrying the extra fat around my stomach."

How did you focus? How important was this to accomplishing your dreams?

"I started experimenting with different foods and ways of cooking, which gave me the passion and drive to stick to my new way of eating. And ever since I started eating the right portions at the right times, I have stopped feeling hungry – which felt great. I stopped craving all the processed carbohydrates that I used to eat, and was happy to be free of them. And I sometimes have a piece of chocolate, as I know it won't sabotage my goals."

What challenges did you face along the way? How did you overcome them?

"Once I discovered I don't digest wheat or gluten very well, going out for meals with my partner became difficult. It's not easy to get gluten free meals at restaurants or cafes, well, tasty gluten free meals anyway! And when I occasionally did revert back to eating unhealthy foods (which usually contained gluten), I felt sick and gained a little weight. This ended up being a good incentive to keep my meals healthy and ask for what I wanted in restaurants."

How did you stay on track with your food when you lacked enthusiasm or faced distractions?

"I prepare my lunch and snacks for work each day, which may seem like a lot of effort, but it's not. It's actually easy and it's a relief to have it ready when I start to feel hungry. It means I don't have to think about every meal and I also know the ingredients of everything I eat. It was hard initially staying away from chocolate and refined cereals, but became easier as I stopped craving those foods. It makes everything so much easier when the cravings disappear."

How did you start and then stay motivated and progress with your exercise?

"I felt that exercise brought me closer to my dad – as though he was watching over me. This got me started and kept me focussed. I started by running three days a week, slowly increasing my running by one kilometre each week. I also did 20mins of interval training twice a week to increase my speed.

I had two personal training sessions a week to learn how to weight train, and monitored my progress with fitness tests and by keeping a note of my running times. This was invaluable for keeping me focussed on my goals.

As my fitness returned, I set targets to reach to keep me motivated. I worked towards running 5km, then 8km and then 10km. I confronted any obstacles head on. I had learnt that we all have challenges to overcome, so I was mentally prepared to find solutions whenever they appeared – and they always do.

I now enjoy every workout and would never turn back! It is part of my life; it is who I am and what I want to be. I am eating healthy food and my goal is now to train for a half marathon - and who knows - maybe one day the Olympics again."

What is the best advice you have for a woman who wants to get into shape?
"Think of your obstacles as challenges. Once you realise you can win any battle, you have the confidence to try anything – no matter how big or small.

Look at yourself in the mirror and really ask the question: "What excuses am I using which are holding me back from changing?" Remind yourself of the person you want to be, as it keeps you focussed on the future and what you can achieve.

Start with some short-term goals and things you know you can change easily. You will be so proud of yourself as you discover your mind and body are stronger than you had thought!

And love your body no matter what shape or size you start out, and with time, it will change. Believe me, it's exciting when your jeans start to feel looser - it really lifts your spirits and keeps you motivated."

Jade's Hot Tips

- Work out what's slowing you down and find a solution so that it doesn't hold you back.

- Deep down you know where you want to go, so make a decision to change - no matter what.

- Don't let any situation or hurdle get in your way and you will achieve anything.

Overcoming Obstacles

"Leaders think and talk about the solutions. Followers think and talk about the problems"
Brian Tracy

Life continually puts challenges in our paths and tests to see whether we have what it takes to overcome them. Whether it's sickness, the death of a loved one, financial stress, work issues, or just busy times – it's how you deal with these experiences that will make the difference. Although we cannot prevent many of life's challenges from occurring, we can control how we deal with them. If we can maintain our health and fitness during these challenges, we are rewarded in two ways. We are able to cope more easily with the mental stresses we face, and we also keep our weight and our fitness on track!

If you face a difficult situation, the best thing you can do for your mental health is to stay physically healthy! Unfortunately, we often forget about looking after ourselves when we most need it. Remember, exercise will give you mental clarity, energy and a good boost of endorphins. A healthy diet will help to keep your moods and energy in check. Good food and exercise will help you sleep.

During these stressful times, lie in bed at night and practice some deep breathing. Keep reminding yourself that staying healthy will help you to cope. Ask a friend to help you stay on track and support you during this time of need.

Resilience

One of the most important assets we can have is resilience; the ability to recover from failures, setbacks or losses. We all come across tough times, but bouncing back after adversity has the most profound impact on our future and its success.

According to Dr. Tian Dayton, a clinical psychologist from the New York Psychodrama Training Institute, some of the attributes of resilient people include:

- They are able to self-reflect – to look at their own thinking, feelings and behaviour and have enough emotional distance to see themselves realistically.

- They separate the past from the present, which allows them to live in today without sabotaging it with unresolved business from the past.

- They find meaning and purpose in their struggle, which is how growth takes place.

- Reaching the summit requires the right attitude and resilience.

Attitude

A positive attitude helps you cope more easily with life's challenges and brings constructive changes as well as success. A bad attitude will always keep you where you are.

Your attitude could be the one ingredient that prevents you from ever achieving your goals. *You* have the choice how you react to every single situation; so choose a positive reaction. A positive attitude also provides motivation and a determination to succeed.

Saboteurs

Have you noticed how down and negative you feel if you are around people with no direction, people who whinge and blame others but do very little about it?

If you are around these people long enough, you will start to behave in a similar manner. You will see the world in a darker shade and your health can even deteriorate. It's time to remove these people from your life, or at least protect yourself from their influence on you.

Excuses

Think about what you say to yourself when you decide not to make a healthy decision. What excuses do you make? Making excuses for your actions or lack of actions is a habit that is hard to break. However as long as you are making excuses, you are not open to changing the way you do things - so you can't expect to get a different result.

Taking responsibility for every action is one of the traits of successful people. They don't blame anyone else for ANYTHING that happens in their lives. They take stock of the issue and find solutions.

How to Beat Any Excuse

A powerful activity is to change "I can't" to "I won't". Often we make excuses by starting a sentence with "I can't do it" (e.g. exercise today, or eat breakfast or whatever you are avoiding).

When you replace "I can't do it" with "I won't do it", you are led to ask yourself the question, "Why not?" Answer this question, and you will usually find the answer really is: "Because I *choose* not to". Then you have a choice to make about whether you will take action.

If you say to yourself: "I won't exercise today", ask yourself, "Why not?" The answer might be: "I won't exercise today because I'd rather make time for a coffee on the way to work".

Honestly address this question, and you may find that you do have the time to exercise after all. If you got out of bed a little earlier, or didn't watch three hours of television at night, you would have time to complete these activities – you have simply chosen not to.

List your excuses, changing: "I can't" to "I won't":

I won't…

_____

_____

_____

Why not?

_____

_____

_____

I won't…

_____

_____

_____

Why not?

_____

_____

_____

Rather than making an excuse as to why you can't do something healthy, such as exercise or prepare healthy food for the day, try turning it around.

Have a look at why you DO want to exercise and eat well. What are your driving reasons? Do you want to get fit or look good in your bikini? Knowing WHY is the key to staying motivated when you feel like giving up.

Fill in your own solutions below.

The reasons I want to exercise regularly are:

_____

_____

_____

When I feel like giving up, I will remind myself:

_____

_____

_____

The reasons I want to eat well are:

_____

_____

_____

When I don't feel like doing it, I will remind myself:

_____

_____

_____

Blast away those excuses every time they enter your thoughts!

Staying Motivated

*"Nobody has to motivate you to do
what you want to do.
You are motivated from within"*
Dr John Demartini

Motivation is defined by www.businessdictionary.com as 'the internal and external factors that stimulate the desire and energy in people to commit to a task, and to exert persistent effort in attaining a goal. It is the energiser of behaviour and mother of all action. It results from conscious and subconscious factors such as the (i) intensity of the desire, (ii) incentive of the goal, and (iii) expectations of the individual.'

In other words, it's a state of mind that moves you from thought into action. So you need to ensure you have a long list of motivators! We all have different motivators and triggers, so think about what yours are. Is it training with a partner, cooking healthy meals or measuring your achievements and progress?

Staying motivated to maintain your new lifestyle will be easier if you put plenty of strategies in place to keep yourself on track.

Keep goal setting
Set short-term and long-term goals with achievable dates. Short-term goals might include booking activities at the same time each week to help you stick to a routine.

Write longer-term goals on your calendar and visit them monthly. You will be surprised at how much you have achieved! Setting deadlines such as entering sports events or completing a nutrition course are simple, tangible strategies that enable you to see exactly where you are headed.

Find a training partner
Exercise with a partner so you can support each other and set goals together. Consider family, friends and like-minded people from your workplace. If you don't have anyone to train with, join a sporting group where other people will be depending on you to turn up to each session.

Having someone to share your journey with will help you to enjoy yourself in the moment. You will discover that the pleasure is in the present, not just in the end goal. For example, cooking healthy meals with the family, joining the local tennis club or attending healthy cooking classes are great activities to connect with people and make your journey to better health more enjoyable.

Establish support from family and friends
Family and friends play an important role in the creation of the New You. Your lifestyle will be changing, so you need to know you have positive influences around you. Let those close to you know of your intentions and ask for their support.

Recruit and spend your time with people who help your cause. Attract and be attracted to people who exude energy; it's both contagious and productive. Saboteurs are destructive, so align yourself with people who are on your side. Your healthy actions will also lead to improvements in others' lives, too!

Measure and refine
Track your progress with measurements, photos and fitness tests. Use your diary to record times for your aerobic training and details of your weight training so you can review your progress and further advance your training. Take photos of healthy meals to see how your eating habits have improved. Seeing tangible improvements will keep your spirits up.

Reward yourself
Be proud of every small goal you achieve – it will keep you inspired to reach the next target. Celebrating your success in a healthy way allows you to sit back and reflect on your achievements. Even a small reward will remind you that you are doing great things for your body, mind and spirit.

Have your goal date on your calendar so you can look forward to the celebration. Perhaps organise a night away, a celebratory dinner, a photo shoot or buy a new dress for achieving your milestones.

Keep motivated by motivating others

Have you noticed that when people achieve their goals, they want to tell the world? They want to shout it from the rooftops, and you will want to do the same. Once you begin this journey, you will be bursting with vitality and energy and you won't be able to resist. You will be inspired to help others, because you know how it's done. You know how to eat well and cook healthy food in a simple way; you feel fantastic and are rid of any ailments that held you back. You can give this beautiful gift to others.

Becoming involved in some way in the health industry is a great way to stay motivated. Volunteer at a local sporting club, or even become a fitness instructor or swimming teacher, and become a role model for others. Simply joining in with your kids' sporting events spreads the healthy vibe.

What you do will change the lives of those around you; your children, parents, sisters, brothers, friends, work colleagues and even your friends on Facebook! You have the power to transform the lives and health of everyone you come into contact with. If you have this kind of purpose, you are energised, satisfied and ready to give to the world. You can achieve things you never thought possible. Now aren't YOU an inspiration?

Now it's your chance to really think about the obstacles and motivators in your mind and your life. If you can explore and discover some reasons behind your inaction, you can find the appropriate solutions. If you realise that you are being held back by your excuses, other people or a lack of internal motivation, you can remove the hurdles and take action. Let's consider your excuses as well as your motivators.

Explore your motivators

Different strategies work for different people, so think about what motivates YOU. What really gets you focused and jolted into action?

Perhaps you are driven by internal motivators, such as the drive to achieve a goal, the desire to succeed, or to demonstrate to those around you what you can achieve.

List your motivators. I am internally motivated to act by:

_____

_____

_____

External motivators are any influences outside you that inspire you to take action. For example, achieving an improvement in your measurements or fitness, setting new goals, or training with someone can all help to keep you motivated. Setting datelines or entering events is also an effective motivator. We are all different, so consider what would help keep YOU motivated.

I am externally motivated by:

_____

_____

_____

Unfortunately we all have some unhealthy triggers or motivators, as well as healthy ones. Perhaps you eat chocolate for a boost when you are tired, or cancel your exercise if you feel stressed.

To change your behaviour, look for healthy actions that you can take instead, when these triggers occur.

For example: When I feel tired I usually reach for chocolate. I will now take 10 deep breaths or go for a 5 minute walk.

Another example might be: When I'm feeling stressed I skip my exercise for the day. I will now exercise for at least 15 minutes if I'm feeling stressed, because I know I will feel better afterwards.

What action can you take to change your response to unhealthy triggers?

_____

_____

_____

Internal Obstacles

Your internal health is integral to your success, and every single woman's body is unique. What you eat, the functioning of all your internal processes and your weight are closely linked, so consider whether all is well on the inside.

Although we cannot physically see our internal processes in action, we must ensure they are functioning efficiently **before fat loss can result.** If your body is dealing with a considerable health issue, it will direct all of its energy to the cause and its healing. Your body will not metabolise fat, but rather hold onto it until such time as the conditions have been resolved.

At some point along the road to better health, all the ladies featured in this book had some internal issues to contend with – elevated levels of unfriendly bacteria being the most common problem. Half the women also had hormonal imbalances.

Our modern-day lifestyle puts up a big challenge to our body and its health. Our bodies and organs are dealing with issues never faced by our ancestors. Digestion is compromised with poor quality foods and additives, and our hormones and organs are under a lot of stress. This can result in all sorts of health problems, as well as weight gain or an inability to lose it.

Your body needs to be physiologically capable of releasing stored fat to be used as a source of energy. A little understanding of some key issues will help you to take any action needed to improve your state of health.

There are five issues we regularly encounter with clients who are struggling to lose fat – they relate to hormones, the adrenals, the liver, digestion and food sensitivities or intolerances.

Hormones
There are a few hormones which play a significant role in determining your body fat levels. If you have an understanding of how they work, you can manage them for ideal results.

Insulin

Insulin is a well known hormone, but what is its relevance to you and your weight?

Your body's main source of energy is carbohydrates, which are broken down into glucose in the blood. An excessive carbohydrate intake will cause blood glucose levels to rise rapidly. Refined carbohydrates lack the fibre that causes the blood sugar levels to rise at a steadier rate.

To compensate for this rise, insulin is secreted into the bloodstream to lower the blood glucose levels. These high levels of insulin prompt the body to store the excess carbohydrates as fat, rather than releasing it to use as energy.

High insulin levels suppress glucagon, which promotes the burning of fat and sugar, and growth hormone, which is required to build new muscle mass.

The sharp rise in insulin levels also leads to a rapid drop in blood sugars, which results in you feeling hungry and craving carbohydrates again soon after you eat. The more refined the carbohydrates you eat, the more extreme the response.

Your body cannot burn body fat if your insulin levels are too high
TIP: Drink water with half a lemon squeezed into it before meals to help regulate insulin levels. The polyphenols in lemons also aid digestion and give you a great vitamin C hit.

Cortisol
Cortisol is the stress hormone made by the adrenal glands. Many of us have such stressful lives that cortisol is constantly being produced. Our stores of this hormone eventually become depleted and this sends a signal to fat cells to store as much fat as possible.

Cortisol also triggers food cravings and overeating. So good stress management strategies are important for good metabolism!

"Whether one's stress is the result of physical or psychological factors, the response mounted by the body's hormonal system is exactly the same"
'The Cortisol Connection'
Shaun Talbott, Ph.D

Oestrogen Dominance

A woman's balance of her main sex hormones is tested throughout her life. As these levels fluctuate, women experience difficulties with weight gain, PMT and issues with the reproductive system. Keeping these hormones in balance becomes more difficult with age and can be exacerbated by chemicals in food and the environment, as well as chronic stress.

The most common problem is oestrogen dominance, which occurs when your body produces or absorbs too much oestrogen. It can cause weight gain and a persistent inability to lose the weight despite eating well and exercising regularly. It seems that no matter what you do, the weight will not budge. The weight usually accumulates around the hips, buttocks and thighs.

Oestrogen dominance is exacerbated by synthetic oestrogens. As well as the necessary oestrogen produced by the body, women absorb synthetic oestrogens, usually through plastics. These man-made chemicals mimic oestrogen in our bodies.

To prevent weight gain from oestrogen, avoid plastics and foods and products containing toxins. Buy organic and free range products to reduce your exposure to pesticides and fertilizers.

It can also help to consume foods that block absorption of oestrogen-promoting substances, such as cruciferous vegetables (see table below).

> ### Tip
>
> Animal products tend to bio-accumulate toxins from their pesticide-laced feed, concentrating them to far higher concentrations than are typically present in vegetables. So ideally, consume organic meat and wild-caught fish to avoid the extra toxins entering YOUR body.

Strategies for Hormonal Balance and Healthy Insides

DO	AVOID
Buy organic and free-range produce	Foods high in toxins and pesticides
Eat more: chicken, eggs, high fibre fruits and cruciferous vegetables (such as broccoli, cauliflower, Brussel sprouts, kale, bok choy, cabbage), whole grains, ground flax seeds, chia seeds and good fats	Sugar, caffeine, alcohol, processed foods, high GI foods and trans fats
Eat wild-caught fish	Farm-raised fish
Include vitamin B complex, C, magnesium and calcium	
Drink lemon juice in water before meals	
Drink filtered water – from a glass	Tap water and plastic bottles
Store and cook foods in glass or ceramic containers	Plastic containers, non-stick pans
Natural cleaning, skin care products and fragrances made with essential oils	Products made with chemicals
Exercise	Inactivity
Get adequate sleep and sunshine	Stay up late and spend too much time indoors
Relax and meditate	Stress

The Adrenals

The adrenal glands are responsible for the production of numerous hormones in the body, including cortisol and a small amount of sex hormones. All these hormones fluctuate with stress.

Your adrenals must manage any stress the body endures. Whether it is physical, emotional, or as a response to ill health, the hormones released by the adrenals are continually tested. If, for any reason, they cannot cope, you will be adversely affected. Your immunity, energy, cravings and physical stress levels will be compromised, as will your ability to lose fat. The adrenals also regulate blood sugar levels, so if they are overworked, cravings and sugar highs and lows will increase and affect your moods, energy levels and ability to lose body fat!

Long-term stress overworks the adrenals, which can lead to adrenal fatigue, a state in which the exhausted adrenals cannot respond adequately. This is a debilitating condition, causing fatigue and depression.

Adrenal and other hormonal gland dysfunction can cause cravings for sweets, weight gain, allergies, heart palpitations, insomnia, depression, fatigue, poor memory, headaches, nervousness, inability to concentrate, recurrent infections and glucose intolerance. To maintain proper adrenal function it is important to control your blood sugar levels, by balancing your meals and eating regularly.

If you think you may need to investigate your hormone levels, a functional hormonal test is the first step. The best test for this is a circadian test, which evaluates fluctuations of the salivary hormone levels over a 24-hour period. The saliva test is seen as more reliable than a blood sample, which only measures total hormone production at the moment of sampling.

The Liver

The liver is an amazing organ which has over 500 functions, including the production of essential proteins and the metabolism of and absorption of fats and carbohydrates. It also eliminates harmful biochemical waste products and detoxifies alcohol, medications, and environmental toxins. It even assists with the digestion and absorption of fats and the fat-soluble vitamins A, D, E, and K.

The liver works hard for you on a daily basis, conquering the toxic enemy of refined carbohydrates, toxins and unhealthy fats. It is the hardest working organ in the body, yet it rarely gets a thank you for its efforts.

Modern lifestyles mean the liver is battling to cope with the role of detoxification, and has little time to manage its other tasks. The breakdown of fat as an energy source must take second place.

We rarely give our liver a second thought, except when it starts to fail. The first sign of this is when the owner starts gaining fat stores, not just around the liver, but in more noticeable places such as the hips and thighs. Secondly, the owner feels unwell or even toxic and may begin to investigate. A continued poor diet and lifestyle will eventually lead to more harmful conditions.

One of the best strategies to make your liver happy is to clean up your diet! This will free up the liver to regulate metabolism and use fat stores for energy rather than dealing with all the added toxins. Also, eat a small meal or snack every three to four hours to avoid becoming hungry. If you are hungry, you have already run out of fuel, which places additional stress on your organs.

Digestion

If you are not able to digest nutrients properly, your metabolic processes will be compromised and malabsorption conditions may result.

Research shows that your intestinal bacteria may also have a big impact on your weight. Andrew Gewirtz and his team of scientists from Emory, Cornell University and the University of Colorado at Boulder, USA concluded: "Our results suggest that people may be eating too much because their appetite is stronger due to changes in their gut bacteria, relative to what someone might have had 50 years ago."

Many of my clients have discovered that imbalances in intestinal bacteria have prevented them from losing weight, no matter what action they took.

For example, sugar will damage your good bacteria, reduce their growth and increase the levels of bad bacteria, yeast and fungi that cause disease. If your body is preoccupied with managing these health stressors, it doesn't have the ability to allow your body to use your fat stores for energy.

If you think you may have a bacterial imbalance, see a naturopath or kinesiologist so they can test your levels of bad bacteria and prescribe natural remedies.

Intolerances and sensitivities

If you have tried various strategies and are still not losing your excess fat stores, the missing key may be that you need to reduce or eliminate foods that cause an irritation. Your body can be sensitive to any food – even healthy foods – which may surprise you.

It can be hard to detect which foods you are sensitive to while they are still in your diet. The negative effects of these foods can be very subtle and you may not realise the affect they are having on your body. They may be preventing you from losing weight or making you feel tired.

If you do not feel like eating first thing in the morning, it may be because your digestive tract is inflamed or not functioning optimally. Once you improve your diet your digestive problems should ease.

If you suspect a food is irritating your digestive tract, eliminate it for three weeks before slowly reintroducing it into your diet again. Undertake this process with one food at a time; otherwise, you won't know which was irritating you!

If symptoms persist, consult a health professional such as a kinesiologist or naturopath. They can test you for food sensitivities and unravel any mysteries surrounding your diet.

The most common irritants to the digestive system are gluten, lactose and wheat.

Gluten

Gluten is a protein in certain grains which can be difficult to digest. Gluten-containing grains include barley, bulgur wheat, durum wheat, kamut, oats (usually contaminated by gluten in processing), semolina wheat, spelt, triticale and wheat. See Step 4 for a list of gluten-free grains and flours.

Bloating and stomach pains are the most obvious symptoms of gluten intolerance. Some people do not tolerate any grains well, so do a little experimenting – there are plenty of other foods which you can substitute. Rice, for example, is usually well tolerated.

Lactose or casein

Lactose is the milk sugar found in cow's milk and is important for infants, not adults. If you think you may be sensitive or intolerant to the lactose in milk, eliminate it for three weeks and then slowly reintroduce it to see how your body reacts. Some people develop lactose intolerance because they have low levels of the enzyme lactase, which breaks lactose down. These people cannot tolerate milk but some can eat yoghurt and cheese. Lactase tablets are available, but this is only a bandaid solution. It is much preferable to eliminate lactose from your diet or choose high quality lactose-free milk. Raw milk is more easily digested and suitable for some people.

Some people are sensitive or allergic to one of the proteins in milk, known as casein. This is more difficult to avoid, as derivatives of casein are used in a wide range of foods. If you are allergic to casein you will probably already be aware of it, as symptoms include eczema, hives and gastrointestinal symptoms similar to those of lactose intolerance and asthma. You could try A2 milk, which is more easily digested if lactose is not an issue.

So if you have a feeling you are not digesting your latte well, look into it…

Wheat

Through great marketing, our addiction to grains and busy lifestyles has led us to rely on wheat as our main food source. Very often, it is eaten for breakfast (most cereals), for lunch (bread) and for dinner (pasta). The excessive consumption of this cheap and irritating grain can result in weight gain – or the inability to lose the fat – and even bad moods.

Investigate any issues that are preventing you from losing fat. For example, if your body is working hard to heal a faulty digestive tract or hormonal imbalance, it will not allow you to lose weight. If you are under a significant amount of stress, it will prevent you from releasing fat as a fuel source. If you free your body to function naturally and efficiently, it will be able to assist you. This is vital to the end goal of permanent fat loss.

Action

Mind...

Think about any internal obstacles you face in your quest for good health, such as a suspected hormonal imbalance, too many toxins or too much stress. Write them down, followed by their solutions.

Obstacle:

_____

_____

Solution:

_____

_____

Obstacle:

_____

_____

Solution:

Body...

Have a good think about the state of your insides – do you need to investigate issues with your hormonal balance, liver or digestion? Make a list and take action if you think any of these needs addressing.

_____

_____

_____

Food:

What foods seem to irritate your gut?

_____

_____

_____

Eat a wide variety of fresh food to aid digestion. Eliminate any foods you suspect are irritating your digestive tract, such as gluten or lactose. Make a promise to eliminate these foods from your diet for three weeks. Then slowly reintroduce them one at a time, and if your body does not respond well, you could be best to avoid them long term.

Keeping Your Mind on the New You

Now that you are on track with the transformation of the New You, it's time to make sure all the strategies you have recruited remain tightly in place.

From this point on, keep on track by continuing the same plan if it's working, and if you learn a more effective way of doing something, then use that strategy. If you step off the track for a moment just get back on it. Change anything that interferes with your vision.

Be different from yesterday. Today is the only thing you can change. Change your mind if you feel like it and refocus on your new plan and a new perspective on life.

Did you know you can have hundreds of thoughts a minute? It's worth letting some of them go - especially the negative ones! Take a deep breath and bring your mind back to your continual progress and how powerful you are.

Make sure your head is clear and regularly ask yourself, "What thoughts are repeating themselves in my head?" Check whether those thoughts are helping or hindering you. Let go of any negative thoughts by not engaging them. If you simply let them flow through your mind without engaging them, they will go away. Take a deep breath and think of something else.

Every day, you can decide to change something about yourself. It might be something small, like eating slowly or thinking about the next day's meal, but it could be something big, such as "I will not engage any negative feelings, I will let them go as soon as those thoughts enter my mind", or "I will change how I view things and remain positive as much as possible". These mind changes are infectious. As you start to be more positive, you will begin to notice how others respond to your new attitude. Just as you will usually smile if someone smiles at you, others will often react positively if you do.

Every day, you will face challenges with family, work and life in general. You can rise above them. You can make any choice you decide to make. You can decide to be successful at achieving your goals, you can decide to feel happy and you can decide to enjoy the process of improving your health. It's up to you.

"Thoughts are always coming and going. One arises, and links with another... The only time they become intrusive is when you engage them. Treat thoughts with indifference, and they'll pass without involving you in any way. Think of them as you would a flow of people past your window. They appear and pass in their own time, but you have no influence or involvement with them. Observe them only in the moment they're passing through. Then let them go..."
Paul Wilson, A Piece of the Quiet, 2007

For more information about programs, eBooks, workshops, cooking classes, free tips and more get in touch or visit us online:

e: info@foodfix.com.au and w: www.foodfix.com.au

Check List

You can use this checklist to track your progress through all the actions you choose to take. Tick them off as you go, to ensure you have covered everything.

Good luck!

ACTION	DONE	NOTES
A. Mind		
Mentally ready & believe in myself		
Seeing the New Me		
Other		
B. Preparation		
Investigated healthy vendors		
Re-stocked pantry & fridge		
Carrying filled snack pack		
Weekly menu		
Prepared meals in freezer		
Cooking extras for next meal		
Other		
C. Health		
More energy		
Better moods		
Lost weight/size/fat		
Less bloated		
Better digestion		
Other		
D. Eating habits		
Eating slowly, fork down		
Sitting down		
Stopping when satisfied		
Never overeating		
Eating when hungry		
Snacking when hungry– the right portion size		
Correct ratio of macronutrients		
Correct meal size		
Other		

ACTION	DONE	NOTES
E. Food changes		
No sugar / less sugar		
No wheat / less wheat		
No dairy / less dairy		
More high quality, living carbohydrates		
Good fats with each meal		
20-30g protein in every meal		
Less additives		
Varied breakfasts– limited cereal		
More organic produce		
Local, high quality produce		
No/less trans fats		
2 litres of water daily		
Other		
F. Exercise		
Sticking to training schedule		
Improving in all areas of fitness		
Changing my goals as I progress		
Fuelling right with training		
Other		
G. Support		
Partner/ family involvement		
Friends/ sporting group or club		
Other:		
H. Obstacles		
Overcome hurdles, excuses		
I. Internals		
Hormones balanced		
Healthy adrenals and liver		
Removed irritating foods		